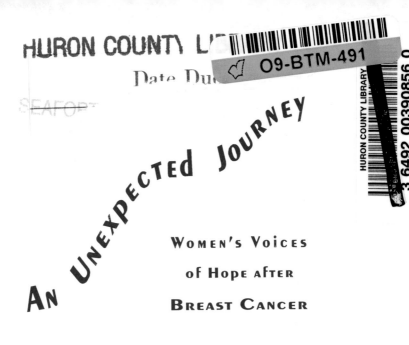

AN UNEXPECTED JOURNEY

WOMEN'S VOICES
of HOPE AFTER
BREAST CANCER

Aniko Galambos

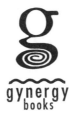

gynergy
books

Edited by: Robert Sean Lewis and Jennifer Lambert
Cover illustration: *The Pilgrimage* by Pamela Pike (from a private collection)
Printed and bound in Canada by: AGMV Marquis

*gynergy books acknowledges the generous support
of the Canada Council for the Arts.*

Published by:
gynergy books
P.O. Box 2023
Charlottetown, P.E.I.
Canada C1A 7N7

Canadian Cataloguing in Publication Data

Galambos, Aniko, 1948-

    An unexpected journey

    ISBN 0-921881-49-5

1. Breast — Cancer — Patients. 2. Breast — Cancer — Psychological
aspects. I Title.

RC280.B8G34 1998   362.1'9699449'00922   C98-950174-4

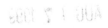

To my mother,
Livia Gotzler, and
to the memory of my father,
Sandor Alex Gotzler.

And to George,
Johnny and Jillian.

Acknowledgements

First and foremost, very special thanks to all the breast cancer survivors across Canada who passionately shared my vision that this book would make a difference, and offered to contribute: Hema Dias Abeygunawardena, Deena Apel, Delores Bartel, Gert Batist, Gwen Binkley, Val Botright, Annette Broomfield, Mary Cloghesy, Rosemary Dankewich, Rev. Sandi Duffield-King, Sister Kathleen Duffin, Sally Gyton, Nancy Herr, Sophie LeBlanc, Beryl MacRae, Gilda Neri, Jill Newfeld, Joanne Paluch, Augustine Pellerin, Elizabeth Potten, Judy Reimer, Chris Sprague, Carolyn VanBuskirk, Jackie Wasserman, Adele and Terry Weir and Brenda Williamson. Their stories matter and I regret that it was not possible to accommodate them all.

My deepest gratitude goes to Robert Lewis, who believed in this book and remained committed to it from the very beginning. Without his wisdom, counsel and technical expertise, *An Unexpected Journey* would not be where it is today.

Thanks also to Eleanor Nielsen of the Canadian Cancer Society and Ann McCallum of the Atlantic Breast Cancer Information Project who spread the word about the project within their organizations.

I gratefully acknowledge Sharon Druker for her generosity in providing legal advice; and all those who read parts of the manuscript and made valuable comments: Imre Ban, Thomas Boczan, Colleen Curran, George Galambos, Livia Gotzler, Tom Sullivan and Saba Zarghami.

I am indebted to my friends who provided various forms of advice and encouragement when I needed it, in particular Sheila Brown, for always being there for me and getting me back on track, and Bonnie Hasan, for unwavering optimism and unconditional devotion. For putting up with my long silences and other idiosyncrasies, thanks to Ethel Major and Emoke Szechenyi.

I also wish to thank Judy DiPietro for being with me at the moment of my diagnosis and sharing my pain; and Carolyn Badger for holding my hand over the past three years.

To George, Johnny and Jillian, thank you for making the sacrifices I asked of you; to my Mom, thank you for being a tower of strength.

Finally, I extend my gratitude to my publishers, Sibyl Frei and Louise Fleming, who made my dream come true, and who faithfully rode the roller-coaster with me this past year.

CONTENTS

Introduction

At three o'clock in the afternoon on February 10, 1994 I changed into my winter boots and asked my secretary to leave everything on my desk. "Claudine, please don't lock up," I said. "I have a report to finish and I'll definitely be back, no matter how late." Rushing down the hall I heard Claudine call out, "Good luck, Aniko." That was the last time I saw my desk, my office, or my shoes.

For over a year I had been putting off seeing the doctor about a lump in my breast. As a senior manager in a national corporation, I was a very busy woman and doctors' appointments didn't fit into my schedule. Now I had no choice. Two days earlier, a needle aspiration had revealed "atypical" cells, and the surgeon wanted to follow up with a biopsy. At four-thirty my worst fears were confirmed. I had breast cancer, and my life changed, forever and irrevocably.

The surgeon didn't intimate that I might die, but like the majority of newly diagnosed women, I understood breast cancer to mean imminent death. My first thoughts were of my family and how my death would change their lives. My husband, George, and I had survived many crises in our twenty-year marriage, but we had done so together. How would one of us manage without the other? And my children! Although they were almost grown — Johnny was eighteen, and Jillian thirteen — they were still my babies. I had so much more to give them. Then there was my mother, a Holocaust survivor who had lost everyone except a sister in the war. She wouldn't be able to endure pain of that magnitude again — the loss of an only child.

The surgeon removed three lumps from my right breast, but he still had "a little more to cut," so I returned to the hospital that evening. In the stillness and solitude of my private room, the initial shock of learning that I had cancer suddenly gave way to rage. I was angry at the whole world — at my husband for not insisting that I quit my job; at my mother for not being more protective of me; at my kids simply for *being* kids, for needing more of my time than I could spare. And most of all, I was angry at my employer for making me sick, for causing me too many sleepless nights over the preceding four years. Ever

7

since my transfer to the personnel department to help "clean it up," my co-workers had seen me as a threat to their elitist culture, undermining my efforts any way they could, and making my work-life unbearable. Now I was paying the ultimate price.

By the time George arrived at the hospital I was so livid that I actually told him I was going to sue the company for giving me breast cancer. "And no matter how things turn out," I continued, "whether I live another two months or two hundred, I will never return to that job. My corporate life is over." I vented like this for almost an hour while he listened, not saying a word. Normally George is an energetic man who walks and talks too fast, who never indulges in an idle moment. Now he was slumped in his chair, his suit looking a size too large, his face pale and gaunt. Seeing him like this sobered me, and I suddenly realized that I needed to become as knowledgeable about this disease as I could. I asked him to go to the bookstore and get me everything he could find about breast cancer.

A few days after my lumpectomy, the books were sprawled across my bed. I didn't know what I was searching for, but still I persisted, moving from one book to the next. To my surprise, my day-nurse advised me to put them away, telling me that I wasn't "ready" for them. I had no idea what she meant, but I knew that they weren't making me feel any better. They were dry and factual, with nothing to say about the devastation I was feeling. Little did I know that the need for a compassionate, human account of the breast cancer experience had already presented itself. *An Unexpected Journey* had been set in motion.

Over the following six months, taking care of myself became my *raison d'etre*. I meditated, practiced visualizations and, of course, underwent chemotherapy and radiation treatments. But I was depressed. I was forty-six years old and suddenly found myself without an identity. Until that point in my life I had been defined by the square-footage of my office-space, the number of windows I had, the direction they faced, the type of wood my desk was made of, the colour of my business cards. In a fraction of an instant these props had been snatched away and I was left with nothing but myself.

I spent the next two years struggling to discover who exactly that self was. Begrudgingly, I came to accept that my past was the result of choices I had made, that if I'd really wanted to I could have quit my job much earlier; with a few small sacrifices the family could have managed on my husband's income. Or I could have gone on to something less demanding, less political, "less" in every respect. I realized that there was no sense blaming the world for my breast cancer, when the truth was that I hadn't been able to let go of the money, the status, and the perks. But with no reason to get up in the morning, no reports to write, no people to deal with nor pressing obligations to fulfill, I felt rudderless. Some people think that quitting my job was a courageous act. It wasn't. I was at the mercy of the pure, raw insistence of my animal soul. I wanted to live. As victims of breast cancer we all do what we must, according to our circumstances and opportunities. For me this meant giving up a career that I knew would kill me.

And then, in the midst of my seemingly purposeless existence I had an inspiration. Remembering the fear and isolation I'd experienced in the hospital after my surgery, I started to understand what my day-nurse had meant about the books I'd been reading. In the intervening months I had educated myself about the science of breast cancer — risk factors, treatment options and the like — but the initial diagnosis would have been much less debilitating had I known personally even one woman who had survived this disease. Instead, the recurring images in my mind had been exclusively of celebrities who had died of breast cancer. It was while reflecting on my own despair that I recognized what I had to do. I would write the book my husband hadn't brought me in the hospital. The one my day-nurse wouldn't have told me to put away. A book about survivors. About hope.

Initially I envisioned writing the book in a question-and-answer format, magazine style, and began by developing a series of interview questions intended to validate the feelings of someone newly diagnosed. How did you handle the "why me" question? Did you make any bargains with God? Did you look for explanations for your disease? Did you think you were going to die? How long did this fear last? Then, questions in hand, all I had to do was find several dozen women willing to go public about their disease and talk openly about their lives!

I had no idea how to proceed, and my approach was unsystematic, ad-hoc, luck-of-the-draw. I began by looking for volunteers through friends and acquaintances, then I'd call people out of the blue, saying: "I've been given your name by so-and-so. I'm a writer who's had breast cancer. Would you like to share your own experience in a book about survivors?" I was nervous every time I picked up the phone. Would they think I was a flake, or that this was some kind of scam? Would they hang up on me?

My worries were unfounded. What I discovered instead was a unique sorority whose members felt indelibly connected to one another and wanted to help in any way they could. If the person I contacted did not feel inclined to participate personally, she would refer me either to someone else or to an organization. Within just a few months I had unearthed a breast cancer network in Canada made up of support and activist groups, as well as various national associations. This made potential participants much easier to find.

I put together a flyer explaining who I was, as well as why and how I was writing this book. And because I believed that an honest relationship between myself and the women was fundamental, I promised each a chance to review and comment on her written story until she was one hundred percent satisfied. I also insisted on using real names, convinced that it would be impossible for readers to identify with a Martha X or a Florence Y. Although this turned out to be an occasional source of delay, difficulty and even exasperation, I was adamant. Real stories required real names.

It wasn't until my session with Sophie LeBlanc — the fourth woman I interviewed in depth — that I realized my initial question-and-answer format wouldn't work. While talking about her medical situation, Sophie and I were naturally drawn to the bigger issues — life, religion, and society — some of which found its way into her story. And from that point on I adopted a different approach. I threw away my questions, letting each woman's life experience determine the focus of her story. I was compelled to write in the first person in order to recount the individual narratives as vividly and directly as I could, as if each woman were speaking to the reader on her own behalf, in her own words, recalling the events of her life just as they had happened. However, in order to ensure anonimity, I have used randomly selected initials to refer to doctors. I have also changed information that would lead to their identification.

I wrote each story immediately after taping it, and was always very anxious when the time came to send it off for its "owner" to review. Although the women understood that their stories were being written in the first person, they had no way of knowing how reading such a text would feel. The stories were theirs, but the words were mine. I had assumed the most intimate of guises — another's voice. Would it ring true? Would she like it? I could never be certain, but I needn't have worried. Their journeys were also mine, and every story grew from that connection. We may have been at different milestones, but we were on the same road, mourning the loss of our former lives; theorizing about what had caused our disease; moving toward a heightened awareness of God, nature, and our proper place in creation.

In my own journey the most rewarding experience has been the writing of this book. I have met some wonderful women along the way — women from diverse backgrounds; from cities as well as small towns; from various races, religions and occupations. Some were diagnosed twenty-five years ago, some thirty-six months ago. And they all shared intimate details about their lives. We would often find ourselves crying together, if a particularly painful memory emerged for either one of us. Frequently we travelled into places they didn't want me to write about — "off the record," they said — exorcising deeply buried demons. They talked about abuse, abortions, drunken families, uncaring or hostile husbands, rejection by their churches and communities. I was always touched when at the conclusion of an interview, *I* would be thanked.

I will never forget when I got on that first plane to do my interviews in the Maritimes. Johnny, who was twenty by then, took me to the airport, and as I got out of the car he said, "Mom, I envy you. You're living a Jack Kerouac-type of life." So I was, and I could hardly believe it myself. Travelling in a pair of jeans with the latest Jane Urquhart novel in my hand, I remember looking with a sense of retribution at the business types nervously reviewing their slide presentations in the waiting lounge.

I travelled from east to west to do my interviews. When I arrived in Charlottetown on the first leg of my travels, I was greeted by The Reverend Sandi Duffield-King, who had invited me not only to stay with her and her husband, The Reverend Barry King, but to conduct all my interviews in their home. Sandi and Barry were models of kindness, and the peaceful and joyous atmosphere of their home made me feel protected and loved. I will never forget the lobster dinner they so enthusiastically prepared for me. For me! Unbelievable.

And in every new city I was welcomed in this loving fashion, invited sight unseen into strangers' lives. In Winnipeg it was Val Botright who left an indelible mark on me. Seeing that I was exhausted after my sixth interview in three days, Val suggested I take a bath, and when I had settled comfortably in the warm water, she entered with a candle in one hand and a glass of wine in the other. "This is how you must relax," she said, before turning off the lights and leaving me alone with my thoughts.

There were many heartfelt moments like these, and I was often humbled by the friendship and trust I received. I had not been aware of a world in which such generosity existed. What a truly great distance I had travelled from my days as a corporate big-shot.

In the course of writing this book, many courageous women have come forward, opening up their lives for me and anybody else to witness. It is unfortunate that only a dozen stories could be accommodated within these pages. However, the twelve stories speak for all of them, and, I believe, for many women living with breast cancer.

We are not leading lives of quiet desperation. We want our voices to be heard so that we can make a difference. And we are counting on the compassion of the human spirit to help move us a quantum leap closer to a cure. Our mothers, daughters and granddaughters — *your* mothers, daughters and granddaughters — deserve nothing less.

Elizabeth Potten

Charlottetown, P.E.I.
Date of birth: October 15, 1944
Date of diagnosis: Summer 1981

What I remember most is the fear. Not my own, but the fear in others — in their voices, on their faces, in their attitudes. And the truth is, even if you have a handle on yourself — or simply believe that you do — when you detect this fear in others, you think, "maybe I *should* be afraid."

I didn't fully appreciate the meaning of "knowledge is power" until the day that I was first diagnosed. Knowledge allowed me to reclaim what was rightfully mine, and what had been confiscated so abruptly from me — my own authority. It put me at the controls of my life, rather than leaving me at the mercy of the medical establishment. Control was my weapon against fear.

Once I had decided to approach my illness in this fashion, I found myself changing, demonstrating characteristics I had never known in myself. I became strong and purposeful, and this became the new prism through which I would experience everything.

In the seventeen years since my diagnosis, I've met hundreds of cancer survivors, and it seems to me that most of us are led by our illnesses into reflection, as if the disease becomes a mandate to alter the course of our lives. I have often wondered why it takes a crisis to lead us into self-examination, but I have no ready answers. Perhaps this is an issue best left to philosophers.

***

My story begins the way, I'm sure, far too many others have. I found the lump while in the shower on an otherwise ordinary summer day in 1981. As I looked for my physician's phone number, I remember staying reasonably calm, but I couldn't keep my hands away from my breast. Maybe I had made a mistake. Maybe if I didn't feel it, just once, it wouldn't actually be there.

My doctor was on holiday, so I was sent to see his replacement. After a thorough physical and a lengthy discussion about my personal and family history, which contained none of the known risk-factors, the doctor was confident. The lump could not be cancerous. "But let's have you seen by a gynaecologist," she said. "Can't do any harm." Off I went to see the gynaecologist.

"No, no. I'm sure it's nothing," he said, "but maybe a surgeon should take a look at you. Just as a precaution." I obeyed.

"Probably nothing," said the surgeon, "but I'd still recommend a mammogram. Baseline. Nothing to worry about." I quickly had the mammogram.

When two weeks went by without any news about my mammogram, I decided to call the surgeon myself. Tracking him down, however, was not a simple matter, and when I finally had him on the other end of the line, he tried to dismiss me, saying he would have called had my mammogram shown anything irregular. I had an uneasy feeling, but let it go. A few days later, the phone rang. He began the conversation by telling me that he had taken another look at my mammogram — which immediately made me doubt whether he had even looked at it in the first place — and that he now recommended a surgical biopsy.

I had the biopsy on October 15, 1981, on my thirty-seventh birthday. The surgeon assured me that I would have the results within twenty-four to forty-eight hours. But when the deadline passed and I heard nothing, once again I had to pursue him. He sounded annoyed — he would not be the last physician to be annoyed with me — and stated dryly that he had not yet received the report from pathology. He pledged to call me the moment it arrived. This is not a man who keeps promises, I thought, so I asked him to get the report right away. I was polite, at least I think I was, but I was also determined. I told him I would stay on hold.

Ten minutes later, he was back on the line asking me to come to his office at once.

I heard myself scream, "bloody hell," but the words never left my throat. And "son-of-a-bitch," was also on the tip of my tongue. Not only had two months of precious time passed since I had discovered the lump, but there had been all those reassurances along the way. Nothing to lose sleep over, they said. Nothing serious. Nothing to worry about. I just couldn't understand it. These people were supposed to be professionals. How could they have been so flippant with my life?

Surely such a series of misdiagnoses wouldn't have happened to an important person, I thought. Therefore, I must not be an important person. And even as I had to absorb the most devastating news of my life, I also had to deal with my own feelings of humiliation. What a sinister combination this was. The gravest insult, however, was doled out by fate. I had spent ten years of my life building up enough courage to leave an unhappy marriage, and had finally done it some ten months earlier. I hadn't even enjoyed one full year of freedom, and now it was about to be taken from me again. Was this it? Was this all I was entitled to — a mere ten months?

On the drive to the surgeon's office, I tried to convince myself to remain rational, take control of the situation, and concentrate on my newly acquired medical knowledge. Thank goodness I had embarked on a massive breast cancer information search the day I found the lump. Many of us believe that we know our bodies best, and clearly my intuition had been more reliable than all the professional "don't worries" I had received.

I entered the surgeon's office intent on being courteous. That's the way I had been brought up. I felt confident, but not defiant. I told him that I had done my research, and that since the tumour was small and — as a result of the biopsy — already out of my body, I was prepared only to have a lumpectomy. I also asked him for the results of my estrogen receptor test. He leafed through the papers in my file and remarked, "It doesn't seem to be here."

"You *lost* it?" I asked. He didn't reply. He avoided my eyes and bent his head over his desk, shuffled some more papers, then reverted to speaking about surgery. But he couldn't disguise his attempt to save face. There were two possibilities: either he had lost the test results or had never requested the test in the first place. I was beside myself.

In the conversation that followed, he insisted that my only option was a mastectomy. He didn't explain why. I knew that lumpectomies were rather rare at the time, but I'm convinced that his refusal to do it was driven by his own needs, not mine. He was afraid of having a black mark against his name if eventually I were to die "on him." And I'm sure he felt threatened because

I came to him well-informed. When I asked him what he would do if I were his wife, he was stunned by the question and probably equally stunned by his answer — which never left his lips.

Ultimately he gave in, although he would not perform the procedure himself. He said lumpectomies were not being done in P.E.I., so he arranged for me to have the surgery in Halifax.

After the operation I was given a clean bill of health. There was no lymph node involvement, and I required no further treatment. The doctors told me to go home and resume a normal life.

It wasn't long before I knew in my soul that this affair was not yet over. I was in a lot of pain, and the healing was slow. Something didn't feel right, and I complained to my local oncologist, whom I had been seeing for regular follow-up sessions. Dr. A. is a warm and kind human being, always generous with her time. Professionally, she was the only one I trusted. I convinced her to refer me to the best specialist within three thousand miles of P.E.I., and a few days later it was done. I had an appointment with Dr. D., a renowned breast surgeon in Montreal.

In the dead of a Canadian winter and armed with my best friend, my X-rays, my slides, my pathology reports, an ice-scraper, a snow shovel, and emergency flares, we set out on the one-thousand-kilometre drive to Quebec in what seemed to be a one-thousand-kilometre-long snowstorm. I remember our hot breath fogging the windshield and how, with my heater acting up, I had to open the windows at regular intervals, the onslaught of stinging snow pounding my face. It was tempting to think that the elements might be portentous.

On the way, we picked up my teenaged daughter, Cathryn, who was working in Katimavik at the time. And as we got closer and closer to our destination, I could sense the fear intensifying in the car. My daughter and my girlfriend weren't behaving like themselves. Idle chatter came easily — bad drivers on the road, a car in a ditch, the snowstorm, the places we were passing — but when I initiated a discussion about the purpose of our trip, their words were sparse and selective, neither of them wanting to let anything slip.

After he conducted a series of tests, Dr. D. didn't take more than twenty minutes to inform me that some serious errors had been committed in my case. There was cancer in the peripheral area of my breast, which had been missed completely in Halifax, and the original tumour, diagnosed as ductal, had, in fact, been micro-invasive. He recommended a full mastectomy.

Although this time it made more sense, I instinctively refused. I told him that I was rapidly losing faith in the medical system and that I wanted to go home to think about it. Dr. D. wasn't pleased. "Just don't take too long," he said.

Actually, what I had said to Dr. D. was a huge understatement. In fact, I really didn't trust doctors anymore. I didn't understand them, and I was struggling to reconcile, in my own mind, the awe they command in our society and what my recent experience with them was telling me. Also, there was a little voice inside my head saying, "Take your time."

I took three months. I set two objectives for myself. First, I wanted to strengthen my body and my mind for the impending operation, and I sensed that a holistic approach would be right for me. I had always been a faithful daughter of the earth and had developed, from an early age, an affectionate relationship with every living thing. So in the months that followed my first Montreal campaign, I began an intensive self-education course on natural healing. I started to eat lots and lots of vegetables and began a strict multi-vitamin regimen that would eventually become my gospel. Not only were these things logical and a natural fit with my disposition, but they were also spiritually satisfying and complementary to my beliefs.

My second goal was to change my entire life — the way I thought, the way I acted and reacted, treated myself, and viewed the world. Of course this wasn't easy, and I often had to remind myself of my own resolve. But the books I read on psychology and philosophy set me on the right path. Norman Cousins had the greatest influence on me at that time, and I followed his example, forcing myself to take humour in earnest. It was quite a challenge to find laughter when grief was so readily available, but, like most things, it was all a matter of practice, and I soon came to acknowledge that humour is the antioxidant of the soul.

Of course, I also had Andrew, my son, to rely on. He was only sixteen, but very mature for his age and always ready to pick me up when he saw "that look" on my face.

As time marched on, my poor oncologist, Dr. A., checked up on me every week. "They're calling me from Montreal," she'd say, with a sense of urgency in her voice. "We want to book you as fast as we can." Or, "Please, Elizabeth, get on that plane." I knew she meant well. Still, I was firm. "Don't push me," I replied. "I'll do this when I'm ready."

I went to Montreal at the end of April. Dr. D. took one look at me and commented that he couldn't believe the difference. He said it was amazing. Given my outward physical appearance — my colour, the texture of my breast — I looked a whole lot healthier than I had back in February.

In retrospect, I should have thanked him and headed for home. I should have told him that I was feeling great and would simply continue doing what I had been doing. Instead, I stayed in Montreal and had the mastectomy. But retrospect is really just a word, isn't it?

***

Victor, my now ex-husband, had been my brother John's best friend when we were growing up, and whenever they would allow, I trailed around behind them. At eighteen, John left home to explore the South Seas, and Victor and I became close friends. He provided emotional support during a period in my life when I most needed it, and since I had not yet given myself a chance to branch out on my own, I'm not surprised that I chose to marry young.

Victor was extremely smart in school, and although he was not quite two years older than me, he was graduating from university at the same time that I was graduating from high school. We got married shortly afterward, in 1963. My daughter, Cathryn, was born one year later, and Andrew a year after her.

It was an unstable marriage from the start, with Victor trying to find himself, doing a little of this and a little of that. We moved three times in five years, from city to city, until he eventually became a high school teacher and we settled in North York. There, I had my first vegetable garden, which opened up an entirely new world to me. But soon Victor got tired of his job and began looking for new horizons. We had some good friends who owned a farm near Dryden and that became our next address. When Victor thought he might like to try his hand at farming, I was delighted.

In 1974 we loaded up a truck with our worldly belongings and went off to the Maritimes. Victor landed a teaching job on Prince Edward Island, and I couldn't have been happier; we had the opportunity to purchase our dream.

The farm we bought turned out to be a magical place. It had been built in the eighteenth century and had known only one previous owner. The land itself was one hundred and fifty acres. Our house, in typical Anne-of-Green-Gables style, had a three-sided bay window on the front and delicately peaked dormers set into gabled roofs with a gingerbread top. All white and green. From our bedroom window, we could see our spectacular white pine, rising well above the other trees that lined the quarter-mile driveway. We raised chickens for eggs and goats for milk. The children, from a very young age, were taught to accept responsibility for certain farm chores and to care for the animals. I thought I would never move again.

Within a few years, Victor had decided to give up teaching and try farming full-time, so I had to find outside employment to supplement our cash flow. First I took on a seasonal job planting trees for forestry. Later, I became a bartender — one of the stupidest things I have ever done, what with all the smoke and alcohol around me. Since I still had my share of the farmwork and sole responsibility for the physical and emotional well-being of the children, this interval in my life was difficult and particularly demanding. In order to get everything done, I rose with the sun and the roosters, put in a full day as wife and mother, went to the bar at five and returned home at midnight. After a few hours rest, the routine would start all over again. I don't remember sitting down once in three years.

Finally, in 1980, six years after we had moved to the Island, we decided to go our separate ways. The farm sold quickly, and the children and I rented an old house, taking some of the animals with us. Victor drove off into the sunset.

Ten months later I was diagnosed. Victor felt that he should return to see me through it, but I told him to get on with his life. I would manage just fine from here. After all, I was not alone.

Cathryn and Andrew had been a great source of strength to me during the separation, and would ultimately be so again throughout my battle with cancer. We have always been kindred spirits, and our ability to speak frankly with each other has been a treasured gift.

**

When I returned from Montreal, life blossomed like hibiscus in the spring. Although Great Revelations About Life coagulated in my brain only after my diagnosis, I had begun to take small steps in the right direction a year or so before that. Still married at the time, I had decided to escape the harmful environment of the bar in order to become a waitress at a resort hotel in Brudenell.

I went back to work a month after my mastectomy, but was soon lured away by the owners of a new restaurant near the Wood Island ferry. The building was a century-and-a-half-old private residence, typical of its time and location, and the owners had taken great care to preserve its antiquity and charm. The restaurant had ten tables and required no more than four staff, two in the dining room and two in the kitchen. The chef was an eccentric gay fellow from Austria and a masterful artist of his trade. His partner and sidekick was actually an ornithologist, a perfect pain, who was self-taught and had a penchant for outrageous desserts with bird themes. I never knew what I would be bringing out of the kitchen from one day to the next. It was a fun place to work, and it was good for me. The ambiance and the camaraderie created an atmosphere reminiscent of the happier times of my childhood, when I had helped my grandfather take care of his visitors at his own grand resort.

I was about ten years old when my grandfather, Bampa, had bought a magnificent piece of undeveloped property in the Muskoka region, about two hundred and fifty miles northwest of Toronto. There was a small, run-down log cabin on the point jutting into the lake, and fifty acres of land stretching from the cabin into the woods. As a child, my biggest pleasure was walking through the trees — so dense, dark and mysterious — enchanted by the narrow beam of light that managed to reach the forest floor. Or I'd escape to the lake and canoe from dawn to dusk in quiet solitude.

Bampa was a natural in the hospitality business, and set out to pursue his dream to build a summer resort in the Grand Hotel style of the fifties. I remember the wonderful times I spent with my brother, watching the unleashed energy of large, sweaty men transform wooded wilderness into a place of pure joy for all of us. At the same time, Bampa renovated the old log cabin on the point. The larger part became our summer cottage; what remained was Bampa's own private retreat.

Once the hotel was up and running, it was teeming with guests who were most appreciative of John's and my efforts to please them. It was a big treat for us to be there with Nana and Bampa on summer holidays, feeling terribly important, helping to clear paths through the woods, cleaning the shuffle-board court, washing cars, or waxing Bampa's old boat.

There was something special about the hospitality trade; I always found self-fulfilment in making others happy, satisfying their needs, and serving them well. That's why working at the restaurant was such good therapy for me. We were one big happy family, living the script of a looney-tunes cartoon.

On the home-front, I continued to live within the context of my breast cancer experience, doing what I had begun in the three months between my two Montreal campaigns. I realized very early on that self-education would be a never-ending process. It was not the physiological aspects of healing that concerned me most. Rather, I delved more and more into the core of natural healing — herbs, vegetables, juices, vitamins, extracts. In my mind the evidence was indisputable.

I should mention that I never blamed myself for getting cancer, nor considered it bad luck. I see it more as the result of the way we go through life, unaware of how the past and the present will affect our future.

Except for the times I had spent with my grandparents, I had not grown up in a happy environment. So, from the beginning, I believed that my childhood and my marriage had been major contributors to my disease. Gradually, however, my knowledge widened and I put equal blame on my life-long exposure to toxins. Out of this grew my passionate belief in the value of all things organic, and I began to grow my own food. Whatever I could not grow on my own, I purchased from reliable sources, even if that meant shipping things in from the other end of the continent. The only items I bought at the supermarket were bathroom tissue, paper towels, and the like.

My longest struggle was with vegetarianism. I loved the farmer's life, and eating meat was an integral part of it. So I manoeuvred around my conflict by continually reducing the amount of meat in my diet. (It would be another ten years before this conflict would be resolved and I would finally give up what had always been an immense source of pleasure for me.)

By 1984 both Cathryn and Andrew were attending university off the Island, and mothering had become a part-time job. In the same year, my divorce became final. I had both time and a clear head to devote myself to volunteer work. Certainly I enjoyed my job and cherished my animals, but I also had an impelling urge to see women become more educated, more aware of their options, and better able to take control of their disease. I became active in the Canadian Cancer Society, helping organize the first chapter of

Cansurmount on the Island, visiting with patients who recently had undergone mastectomies, making myself available whenever and wherever there was need.

Medically, I had never felt better. My only problem was the plastic prosthesis I had been wearing since the mastectomy two years earlier. It was very uncomfortable and wouldn't stay where it was supposed to. Feeling overconfident because of my good health, I decided to consult a plastic surgeon. An implant would be particularly useful in my situation, I was told, considering that waitressing and working with farm animals both required heavy lifting. It would restore my body's natural balance. But I was hesitant and needed to be convinced. On my third visit to the plastic surgeon, I opened the door and announced, "I'm ready."

"I'm so glad," the doctor replied. "It is certainly the right decision for you."

I went ahead with the silicone breast implant in February 1984. Of course we all know what a terrible mistake that would turn out to be.

***

Meanwhile, my work as a volunteer was about to take me in a direction that I never could have anticipated.

One day the conversation at the restaurant turned to cancer. Francesca, my co-worker, knew that I had had breast cancer and was aware of the volunteer work I was doing with the cancer society, so she didn't feel uncomfortable broaching the subject.

She told me that during a small dinner party the previous evening, a friend of hers — a doctor, in fact — had been lamenting the sorry state of palliative home-care on the Island. He had a patient in the final stage of cancer whose only desire was to go home to die, but since there was no infrastructure on P.E.I. to accommodate such a wish, there was nothing he could do for her. An emotional discussion had ensued with the doctor finally suggesting that they start a hospice on their own.

At this point in her story, Fran looked at me eagerly and proposed, "Elizabeth, why *don't* we?"

I didn't need long to think about it. It was a natural next step in my evolution, and there was something about dealing head-on with death that attracted me.

Within days we were off and running. Having our hearts in the right place, however, was clearly not enough. Our first and biggest challenge was to learn the business of hospice care — the practical, organizational, and operational aspects. We successfully applied for a Canada Works Project grant, and this gave us the start we needed.

In the process of establishing the Hospice of Southern King County, Inc., we quickly found out that information on this subject in North America was sparse. It was 1984-85, and the AIDS movement as yet had not been conceived (AIDS was relatively unknown or, if known at all, was considered a strictly homosexual affliction.) And the notion of hospice care was alien, even scary, to a society that had always sidestepped death.

At the time that we were starting out, I had already made plans to visit my daughter's new in-laws in Holland. And I thought that once I was over in Europe, I should go to St. Christopher's in London — reputed to be one of the best hospices in the world. I spent several days helping, learning, and gaining experience. I collected volumes of literature, books, studies, videos, and every other type of material I could buy or borrow from St. Christopher's. I still recall the exorbitant price of the excess-baggage weight and how the Canadian customs officer, upon inquiring about the nature of my business, brusquely waved me through.

No sooner had I arrived home when Fran and I began to feel the enormous demands of our undertaking. We needed to develop training programs for volunteers and family members of terminally ill patients. We had to organize seminars and do a lot of P.R. work to educate the public, all the while learning about hospice care ourselves. Most importantly, we were immediately called to task. Fran's first patient was the woman whose wish to die at home had originally inspired us in this direction. My first visit was with a 63-year-old man who, the day before his passing, had walked to his mother's house on his own two feet to say goodbye. It was at his bedside that I understood, for the first time in my life, the true meaning of courage.

Within a year, the hospice evolved into a self-sustaining organization staffed by dozens of volunteers. Fran became its coordinator and sole paid employee, and I stayed on as Chairman of the Board. My formal involvement lasted the better part of four years. As a footnote, the Hospice of Southern King County celebrated its thirteenth anniversary this year and is continuing to grow, thanks to the immense dedication of people in the community.

In the meantime, unbeknownst to me, the man who would become my second husband had entered my life. Gordon and I had known each other for some time and had enjoyed many refreshing early-morning walks together in the salubrious Island air, our panting boisterous dogs circling around us. We considered ourselves good friends, nothing more. And I was happy with this relationship.

Then, in 1987, this began to change. My son, Andrew, was heading out to the California Institute of Technology for graduate studies. It was his intention to drive there, so in his last year of undergraduate school, he took a part-time job to finance the purchase of a car — a 1969 MG classic that won his heart. Despite what it cost him, the car required serious repairs, and he spent all summer trying to get it ready for the trip. Then time ran out on him. He ended up flying there, and we enlisted Gordon to help complete the work.

When Andrew's car was ready in the fall, I decided I would drive it to Victoria, visiting my best friend at the same time, the woman who had accompanied me on my first trip to Montreal and had recently moved west. Andrew flew up to join me for Christmas, and shortly afterward we headed back to California, making our way through the narrow, winding fissure between mountain and ocean that is the old coastal road. What a memorable trip that was, indeed.

In California, I, too, became smitten with sports cars and bought myself a 1967 Alpha Romeo, which would also become my transportation home. Andrew kept saying, "Gordon will *really* love this car." Luckily, it behaved well during the mammoth trip, showing signs of fatigue only when I drove off the Borden ferry. I asked Gordon if he'd be interested in doing the work on it, and he jumped at the chance. He was an old-car buff himself and Andrew turned out to be right. My relationship with Gordon really developed from there. We got married three years later.

In the summer of 1991 Gordon and I purchased a twenty-seven-foot motor home, which became our residence-on-wheels. We would spend six months of the year on the Island and six months in the southern United States. It was during one of these trips to the U.S. that problems with silicone breast-implants first made headline news.

We were lucky to be in the States when this issue blew wide open. Detailed information became immediately available, and there was plenty of it. For weeks, revelations about silicone implants were the top item on the evening news, which often contained special reports and lengthy interviews with scientists, doctors, and the like. Of course lawyers were quick to get in on the action too, and 1-800 ads, with promises of instant wealth, burst across the media like daffodils across landscapes in May.

Those who were unaffected shook their heads in disgust. Victims panicked. As for me, I had been experiencing pain in my left side for quite some time, and now recognized that it was my own implant screaming, "Let me out of here!"

Research expedition, round two, began. I gathered newspaper clippings, scientific articles, medical journals, videotapes of television-magazine shows, and photocopies of anything even remotely connected to implants. There were papers all over our motor home — two-foot-high piles on the table, on the chairs, and even under the chesterfield. Walking about was like stepping on stones in a river. Gordon turned to me one day and said, "Never in my life did I think I would have looked at so many breasts."

When we arrived back on the Island in 1992, I immediately went to see my family physician, insisting on a complete series of tests. I had developed neurological problems by then, was generally in ill-health, and was sure that either the cancer was back or my implant was leaking. Except for an irregularity my oncologist picked up, the results of all my tests were negative. It was not until a second battery of tests, one year later, that a needle aspiration finally confirmed a new malignancy. There was cancer in my other breast.

Instead of running straight into a surgeon's scalpel, I resolved to strengthen myself again, the way I had done twelve years before. However, I first needed to know what I was dealing with, so I looked for confirmation that both my cancer and my neurological problems were silicone-related. I contacted the leading breast-implant specialist in North America, who provided me with enough information to convince me I was right.

Although I was anxious to have the silicone breast-implant removed, I couldn't find a doctor who would be willing to do it on my terms. I wanted to remain conscious during the procedure, and asked that it be performed with only a spinal block. I was very worried about the general anaesthesia. My neurological problems, my overall ill-health, and the two previous bad reactions that I had had to it led me to believe that I would never make it out of an operating room alive. My thoughts were incomprehensible to medical people. I left them speechless and in obvious fear for my life. And they put this down in writing. I was on my own.

To start my rehabilitation, I first had to ensure that I would do no further damage to my system. It was at this point that I completely dedicated myself to vegetarianism. I eat strictly organic foodstuff now, most of which I grow myself. Broccoli may look nice on the shelf, but I simply don't trust anything that comes from a store.

Then I set out to detoxify my body. This wasn't just a matter of expunging the silicone that was leaking everywhere inside. It was about getting rid of all the toxins my system had accumulated since childhood. Take DDT for instance. As a youngster, it had been my job to spray the screens on our summer cottage, and I remember how much I enjoyed doing it, inhaling as I went from window to window, breathing in its lovely, floral perfume. Then there was Brantford, where I grew up. Brantford is an industrial city, with an asphalt plant and a rubber plant. On my way to school each day, tall chimneys stood erect in my line of vision, like rooks on a chessboard. The sight of smoke rising to join the clouds was enchanting to my eyes. And the Grand River was so polluted back then that we could neither swim nor boat in it.

Today, my detoxification regimen often includes a three-day fast using fermented vegetable juices. Beet juice, in particular, is a known tumour-re-ducer. I also take essiac and a specific combination of vitamins. For example, during the course of a day, I will consume sixty tablets of Vitamin C, 500 mgs. each. I drink a lot of herbal tea and there is a special green food drink I buy from a Vancouver supplier that contains spirulina, chlorophyll and a variety of herbs. I am on a path of continuous education because there are new things coming out in this field all the time.

Over the years, Gordon and I have worked very hard to enable ourselves to live according to my way of thinking. We've built a large greenhouse — 32 x 18 feet — and this allows us to extend the growing season from an average of six months to nine. Friends on the Island supply us with organic wheat, and anything else I may need comes from carefully researched, reputable sources. As you can imagine, this lifestyle keeps us pretty tight financially.

It is my strong belief that if I listen to my body each day and nourish it, as well as my mind and soul, my life will be complete whether I live for a week or another fifty years.

Afterword

Today, my life is as beautiful as I could wish it to be. Andrew received his Ph.D. in mathematics and is currently teaching in England. Cathryn moved back to the Island after obtaining her business degree, and started a media graphics business with her husband. Often, when I look at her mothering her two small children, I can't help but giggle. Now it's her turn, I think to myself. Now she gets to do what I had to do for so many years, while I sit back and enjoy being a grandmother.

I still have the cancer, which drives my doctors crazy, and I still have the silicone breast-implant.

I have been very fortunate to meet, fall in love with, and marry the most kind, generous, and loving person on this earth. Our relationship is a very happy one. We are in complete control of our lives and, indeed, live the motto, "one day at a time." Although we are no longer travelling, we continue to live in our motor home and are in the process of building a small log house, reminiscent of my grandfather's private retreat in the Muskokas. That's where we'll retire, because with Gordon by my side, I plan to be around for a good long time.

If you are ever in our neck of the woods — and I assure you it is well worth the trip — do drop in for a cup of tea. It is easy to recognize our place from the main road. Immediately after you see the mailbox that looks like a miniature log house, make a left into the woods onto a narrow, secluded road.

When our friends come to visit, making their way along the forested driveway with its magnificent steeples of pine and spruce, they say that they can actually feel the peace.

Beryl MacRae

Charlottetown, P.E.I.
Date of birth: May 16, 1945
Date of diagnosis: June 21, 1993

I should begin by telling you that my breast cancer experience has been rather ordinary — except, perhaps, for the extraordinary fact that I have had it. But sadly, even this is becoming a much too common occurrence these days.

I have not been reborn as a result of my experience, and I am not one of those women who can claim it is the best thing that has ever happened to her. For me breast cancer was a journey through pain, with personal disappointments along the way. I can admit these things now because I'm much stronger than I used to be. I don't think anyone can survive this ordeal and remain untouched by it. So my story is also about my personal growth, new achievements and, for better or for worse, a different way of looking at the world.

I was forty-eight years old in the spring of 1993 when a routine mammogram showed a suspicious cyst. That was how it started.

My doctor was cautious as he gave me the news, saying the cyst was likely benign and that it only needed to be drained. So I quickly went for a needle aspiration. When it was over, I remember feeling extremely relieved, thinking that was the end of it. But a few days later the cyst had filled up again. I went back for another needle aspiration, and this time the fluid had a pinkish hue. My doctor immediately referred me to a surgeon.

One week later I was in the surgeon's office, stoically listening to the three options he outlined for me. I could go home and forget about the whole thing (which, admittedly, he did not recommend), I could have the cyst drained again, or I could undergo a surgical biopsy. Dr. G. didn't appear too concerned, and I was caught completely off guard by the idea of a serious intervention, so I decided to have yet another needle aspiration. This time the contents were sent out for analysis.

I spent an anxious couple of days waiting for the results, aware that the lump was filling up again. But when I went back to see Dr. G., he was calm and confident as he read my pathology report. There was nothing to worry about, he said. The results indicated that the lump was, indeed, benign and now it was a perfectly viable option for me to go home and put everything behind me.

Of course his words were very appealing, but logic led me in the opposite direction. This lump had not always been there. It was not natural and had no function in my body. And although I felt uncomfortable disagreeing with him — questioning a surgeon's judgement was a foreign notion in my book — I knew I had to speak up. I didn't want to live with doubt for the rest of my life. And so, I requested that he perform a biopsy. To his credit, Dr. G. was very accommodating and appeared to be genuinely sensitive to my concerns.

I went into the hospital on June 14, 1993, armed with numerous reassurances. My family doctor said it was a good sign that no calcifications had been found on the mammogram. There was no history of breast cancer in my family and, all told, I had a lot going in my favour. The surgeon's opinion was similar — less than a one percent chance of the worst-case scenario.

Seven days later, on my way to the surgeon's office to have my biopsy stitches removed, my biggest worry was whether or not this would hurt. I greeted him with a smile, relieved that this visit would mark the end of my troubles. Immediately, I was struck by Dr. G.'s sombre reserve. "I'm afraid I have some bad news for you," he began. And at some point in the ensuing five minutes, I was told that I had breast cancer.

Probably an automatic reflex, my initial concern was to behave in an appropriate fashion and to preserve my dignity. How was I to react? I was a wife and mother, I had a responsible job, and I was a member of good standing in my church and community. This diagnosis suddenly turned me upside down. I was stunned, trying to sort out every thought in my head, when the surgeon declared, "You know, Mrs. MacRae, it's a good thing we decided to do the biopsy."

Well, I couldn't believe my ears! This time, within a blink of an eye, I reminded him that after the test result had come back negative, *I* was the one who had requested the biopsy. He, on the other hand, had confidently advised me to go home. To forget about the whole thing. "I *couldn't* have said that," the surgeon protested. So I quoted the very words he had said to me. Dr. G. succumbed to his conscience, looked directly into my eyes, and said, "In retrospect, that was wrong."

This circuitous apology was my induction into a new world order that would henceforth rule my life. A place where cancer was king and doctors were gods. Where the old Beryl MacRae was dead. In this world I would be someone who was talked about when my back was turned, someone pitied, the poor, unlucky soul, the one out of nine. I would become a line of data in a compilation of health statistics, a truncated sentence on the evening news.

The surgeon didn't waste much time elaborating on the process that lay ahead, and I found myself in a most precarious position. I had just been told I had cancer. What I needed was permission to absorb the news, time to accept and understand what was happening to me. Instead, I was asked to make the most traumatic decision of my life. I had to choose whether or not I should keep my breast. If I kept my breast would I die? If I sacrificed my breast, would that give me a 100 percent guarantee? What if my fate was sealed either way?

I know it was not the surgeon's intention, but by drawing me into this issue on the heels of such a devastating diagnosis, he only made things worse. I had no idea what to do. Like most women, I didn't know much about breast cancer. What's more, I found myself having to deal with this alone. I hadn't asked my husband to come with me that day because I was only expecting to have my stitches removed. I hadn't anticipated anything like this.

Take a hold of yourself, Beryl, I thought. There was a discussion to be had and a decision to be made. In the end, I chose to have a lumpectomy, with the caveat that if the surgeon saw the need to go further during the operation, he had my consent. To me this seemed the most reasonable route. We agreed.

I left Dr. G.'s office and began the long, lonely walk to the parkade, my mind whirling. Normally, the first day of summer was filled with renewal and promise, but now I was wondering what the new season held in store for me. Walking toward my car, I felt my body weakening, and I was somewhat uncertain about my ability to drive. But I got into the car and headed for home. I'm convinced it was neither luck nor my good driving skills that got me there safe and sound. God was in the back seat and controlling the wheel.

Once I arrived home I began to prepare dinner, and rehearsed the lines I would repeat to my family. Everyone came home separately that evening, and I had individual conversations with each of them — my husband, my twenty-three-year-old daughter and my twenty-five-year-old son. Later, I called my mother and told her over the telephone. It was easier that way. To this day I don't know which of the five of us found the news most difficult to take.

That was a restless night, the first of eighteen to follow. The next morning I called my supervisor to tell her about the diagnosis. I also said that I would like to take the day off, and asked her to tell my co-workers so that it would be easier for me to face them the following day.

Thursday, July 8, 1993: The eve of my surgery had finally arrived. Surprisingly, I was not nervous. Quite the contrary. I lay in my hospital bed acutely aware of my environment, secure in the knowledge that soon the cancer would be out of my body. Late in the evening, a nurse came into my room and handed me the consent form. Naturally I took my time reading it, studying it and examining every letter of every word, because this would be the most important paper I would ever sign.

Then I saw it. The description of the surgical procedure read "mastectomy." Immediately my fragile confidence was shattered. I was not familiar with the hospital's practices. I wondered if the consent form was only routine, intended for my file, or if it would be presented to the surgeon before the operation. I had visions of him seeing my signature on the form and thinking, "Oh, she must have changed her mind." I called the nurse and was almost apologetic in telling her about the mistake. She was very gracious and returned with a corrected version, but this didn't appease me. I worried all night.

I got through the surgery without incident, and six days later I went home.

By way of testament to a new life after breast cancer, some women quit their jobs or enter the workforce for the first time. Some leave their husbands or make a permanent commitment to a relationship. There are women who climb the highest mountain peaks, the way a group of breast cancer survivors did in Argentina four years ago. My own aspirations were more modest.

On the Saturday following my homecoming, the CP hotel was hosting the Island's annual rose show. I had never seen it before; there had always been something more important to do. Besides, I'd always thought the roses would be there the next year, and I could see them then. But this time I had different thoughts. So I called my mother, she brought a friend along, and off we went to "smell the roses." I had never realized what truly glorious creations they were. And for a sliver of time, all seemed right with the world.

The end of July brought my first appointment with the oncologist and the beginning of my treatments. It was decided that I would have six months of chemotherapy followed by four weeks of radiation.

At the treatment stage of the cancer process, the most important person in our lives is the oncologist. By virtue of their medical training, our oncologists are the only ones who can imagine what we are going through. When we are suffering from the effects of the chemo, only they can validate our pain, and we need to hear the words, "I know. I understand."

We don't ask for friendship. It isn't even necessary for our oncologist to like us. What makes this doctor important is knowledge. The oncologist can make sense of everything that is happening to us and relieve our anxiety, convince us with authority that good will come from bad, that it is a good thing when we enter the hospital feeling well, only to become ill before we leave. We need this person on our fearful journey into the unknown, where we become captives to chemo's omnipotent rule. Unfortunately, my own oncologist understood nothing of this.

During those eighteen fretful days of waiting, the interval between my diagnosis and my hospitalization, I had come across a little five-dollar book called, *The Well-Informed Patient's Guide to Breast Surgery*. It certainly wasn't a Dr. Susan Love-type tome, but to a novice like me it was a good overview of many breast cancer issues, including the different possibilities for post-surgical treatment. When I went to meet the oncologist, I brought the book with me, intent on showing my initiative, that I was ready to become involved in my own recovery. I had read that this was the right thing to do, and anticipated that it would help us get off to a good start.

I did not know this man. My knowledge of him was limited to what a friend had told me — that his parents were lovely people. But to my dismay, that first visit was a disaster. The book, along with my enthusiasm, had exactly the opposite effect. He saw it in my hand and snapped, "Oh, I probably don't have to tell you anything." I was crushed.

This statement turned out to be a vivid reflection of his detached approach throughout the entire course of our relationship. He had never been trained in, nor was he interested in, the humanitarian aspect of disease treatment. He perceived his role as purely technical, and all of our subsequent conversations would be limited to that.

I have gone over this many, many times in my mind and have come to the conclusion that perhaps Dr. J. felt threatened because I came to him inquisitive, not deferential. Whatever the case, a doctor with his indifference should be in pathology, or in a research lab where he can do no psychological damage to his patients. Such a physician has no business dealing with humans, who become even more emotionally ravaged by this callous attitude.

For a long time I meant to tell Dr. J. how I felt. Approximately two years after my treatments had ended, I finally summoned up the courage to do so. I wrote him a letter in the fall of 1995 and held nothing back. My letter concluded as follows:

"I am enclosing information that I found in one of the several books I have read. It is my hope that you will place it in a prominent place in your office as a regular reminder of how a cancer patient would like to be treated by her oncologist. My purpose in writing this letter is the sincere hope that it will benefit other cancer patients who come into contact with you. As far as helping me, it is too late for that. I feel lucky that I have come this far in spite of my negative experience with you."

***

My luck with oncologists did not improve. When I met with my radiation oncologist for the first time, I was shown into a room and told to strip to the waist. No one gave me a hospital gown. I was sitting half-naked on the examining table — but feeling 100 percent exposed — when the oncologist entered in his starched, immaculately pressed white lab coat and sat down on a stool in front of me. He opened the manila cover of my file and began to read to himself while I remained unclothed, watching and waiting. The balance of power was immediately established.

The next thing I knew he was making marks on my chest with what looked like a felt-tipped pen. He explained nothing about the radiation process or its possible side effects. The only thing he said was that I would not be allowed to take any baths. I naturally assumed this had something to do with the effectiveness of the radiation, but I was wrong. It was to preserve the markings on my breast in order to save the oncologist from having to redraw them, in case they became smudged. I later learned that this is a routine advisory for all patients and, of course, I understand. I have no quarrels with it. What I object to was being made to live in constant fear of a drop of water falling accidentally on my breast, thinking that this would undermine my treatments.

Radiation started in February of 1994 and lasted four weeks. And I got stuck with this oncologist every day for the next twenty days.

Despite my physical discomfort toward the end, my husband believed a holiday would be good for me. So when I walked out of the clinic for the twentieth and final time, we got straight into the car and headed for the ferry, then drove down the coast to Myrtle Beach, South Carolina.

The vast open spaces and the fresh air soothed my senses. I felt as if nature were patting me on the shoulder saying, "There, there. It's all over. See the beauty around you and forget about the past." I *did* want to forget, almost everything and everyone, but not Cecilia.

***

I had met Cecilia (we used to call her Cece) through work. She herself had been diagnosed with breast cancer several years earlier. At the time of her ordeal I was so engrossed in my life that I never truly appreciated what she was going through. However, following my own cancer diagnosis, Cece was selfless and determined to help me, and we spent a lot of time talking together. In each instance, Cece gave generously of her knowledge and experience.

I vividly recall one particular Sunday, shortly after my chemotherapy began, sitting on our porch on a sparkling, windless Island afternoon, drinking iced-tea. Cece gave that time, usually spent with her husband and two little girls, to be with me. She told me everything about chemotherapy that day. And just to illustrate how insidious it can be — but never forgetting the importance of finding laughter in every human experience — she

lightheartedly told a story she had heard about a survivor named Ann. It went
something like this:

About a month or two after her chemotherapy had ended, Ann and her
friend, Sheila, organized a night out with their husbands. Throughout
the course of her illness, Ann had been very brave, maintaining an
exemplary positive attitude. To all appearances, she had sailed through
chemotherapy, never complaining, running the household better than
ever, and even making some big changes in her life, such as quitting
her high-level, but stressful job. The movie they went to see was *The
Madness of King George*, not exactly the eighteenth-century costume
drama they had anticipated.

There was a recurring scene in which poor, crazy King George was
tied to a chair, hands behind his back, feet in shackles. He was fed in
this chair, slept in this chair, and even had to relieve himself there.
Halfway through the film Ann began to feel ill. She took a couple of
deep breaths, but it didn't help. In her last moment of consciousness,
she whispered to her husband, "Take my purse, I'm going to faint."

Her husband supported her arms, and they made it out of the
crowded theatre. When Ann came to, she was lying on the carpet in the
hallway, looking straight up at Sheila, who tried to diffuse the situation
by promptly telling Ann that "she looked like hell." Sheila's husband,
never one to let an opportunity go by, said that he had been thinking
about leaving in any event, but couldn't have come up with such a
spectacular exit.

Ann had never fainted in her life, and this incident began to bother
her. She sought out an old friend, a psychologist, who confirmed that
the parallel between what she had seen on the screen and her own
chemotherapy treatments had probably caused her to faint. Like many
women, Ann had taken her treatments in a chair, her arm bound to the
armrest, her hand taped to the IV, helpless, like King George. "So much
for positive attitude," Ann said, then advised her entire breast cancer
support group never to rent the video.

After recounting this story, Cece turned to more practical matters and
handed me the scarves she had worn when she lost her hair. "It's easy," she
said, teaching me little fashion tricks for making stylish turbans. In fact, it so
happened that I didn't lose my hair. It thinned out, but I could still have it
styled rather nicely by my hairdresser.

On other occasions, Cece told me about her own experiences with people, all of which I can now attest to. There are those who will avoid us, scared off by their reflection in our eyes. There are those who will refuse to talk about our illness or listen to our feelings. Others insist on talking only about themselves, the "poor me" types whose daily problems are always worse than our own. And then there are people who are simply insensitive. We agreed that these "toxins," as we called them, should be cut out of our lives. Of course we also agreed that this is easier said than done.

Cece talked about the importance of treats, of rewarding ourselves, and I followed this advice to the letter. For example, to celebrate the end of my chemotherapy, I had a marvellous pina colada party with my other grey-haired friends — the Golden Girls. We drank and sang, and it felt good to laugh again. But my biggest treat to myself was a twin-stoned, sky-blue sapphire ring that I bought on a whim one day, passing by a jewellery store. I never take it off. It is a perpetual reward, because every time I look at it, I am reminded that I'm still alive.

Cece and I talked about family. As women, we have been brought up to be strong. Our primary place is in the home, not merely for doing the chores, but for being nurturers and caregivers. Our families revolve around us, and it is our basic instinct to protect them. They are dealing with their own fears and concerns about our disease, and we don't want to make things worse. Inevitably, we protect them from our pain, our emotional vulnerability, and the worst of our imaginations. We pretend that everything will be all right. We try to maintain a routine in order to provide stability. We make breast cancer a peripheral issue when it is, in fact, the centre of our universe. Cece convinced me that it was okay for supermom to go on vacation, that it was even okay to take an extended leave of absence. We do it for ourselves and, in doing so, we do it for our families.

Cece was a constant source of inspiration to me, and I don't know what I would have done without her.

***

Almost five years have passed since my diagnosis. Overall, my emotions are less intense than they used to be, but there are still times when the feelings suddenly rise to the surface, and I experience the trauma all over again, in full force. As part of my own healing process, I've given a great deal of thought to understanding why these feelings exist and what I can do to master them.

I've read at least a dozen books on breast cancer and found some truth in all of them. But the sentiment I most identify with relates to the overriding feeling of sadness we experience, mourning the loss of our previous lives. As women with breast cancer, we immediately lose a sense of ourselves, and, what's even more disconcerting, we face a potential invalidation of our pasts. Did we get sick because we did all the wrong things? Having lost our former identity, we wander in limbo, struggling to create a new one. Surviving this transition can be an overwhelming challenge, fraught with loneliness and despair. I know this well.

I have also learned that we cannot derive our strength entirely from within. Although it certainly helps to have faith and "a positive attitude," our fundamental need is for human contact. That is our elixir. Family and friends, neighbours and colleagues, members of our church and community all have the ability to either nourish our spirit or starve it. Women who reclaim their lives quickly are fed a continuous diet of all that is good in human nature, from something as seemingly trivial as an acquaintance crossing the street to say hello, to an act requiring a little more effort, such as taping a PBS special on tamoxifen. These gestures of human kindness make all the difference.

I remember the caring nurses at the oncology clinic with much affection. Although I came to dread the chemo itself, Cathy did her best to make it as easy as possible for me. She never inserted the IV tube without saying, "sorry." That small gesture meant a lot to me. I can also recall the time a neighbour brought food to our house and how guilty I felt accepting it. Later I realized that people choose to express their concerns in different ways. One day our daughter returned home with such a huge supply of bread and rolls that I thought she had raided Sobey's bakery. In fact, my sister-in-law had baked them for me.

Behaving as if our disease does not exist will not make it so. We crave compassion, empathy, and understanding. And as true as this is, I recognize it may be asking too much from those who have not walked in our shoes.

Afterword

My breast cancer journey was a difficult one, and it didn't end in Myrtle Beach. Physical problems continued to plague me. Two years ago, I developed lymph edema, and the various treatments I have tried have all failed. Sometimes it is merely uncomfortable; other times recurring infections prevent me from going to work. But I live with it, and try not to complain too much.

I've also had three additional scares. The first lump was biopsied on the Island through a needle-localization procedure, a lengthy and most agonizing process. I later found out that this is generally done under local anaesthesia, but I wasn't given one, and to this day I have no idea why. So when I had my second scare, three months after the first, I decided to research my options. I discovered that a core biopsy procedure was being done in Halifax, and I arranged for a referral. A core biopsy is painless and non-invasive, yielding the same result as a surgical biopsy. Within a week I received the news that the suspect lesion was only fibrosis. Most recently, in February of 1997, another suspicious lesion found on my mammogram also turned out to be benign. Unfortunately, after a positive cancer diagnosis, being afraid becomes part of your life.

However, in spite of these setbacks, I am well on my way to psychological recovery. I can tell you with reasonable certainty that we all recover eventually. But we must all have someone to talk to, someone who will be there for us when the trauma is too great to handle on our own.

I was lucky that I had the support of a wonderful friend in Cece. On December 20, 1995, the metastases with which she had been diagnosed defeated her, and Cece moved on to a more peaceful place. I miss her and think of her often, especially when I have the opportunity to reach out and help someone else, the way Cece reached out and helped me.

Certainly, my breast cancer experience has given me new insight into human nature, and my sensitivities have changed. I spend more time with positive people, with people who replenish, rather than deplete, my energy. And I have made significant changes in my life. The first was cutting back on work. I was lucky that my employer, the federal government, agreed to my request for a four-day week. I have every Friday off now — I call it my "goof-off day." It is reserved for doing only things I enjoy, such as going out with the Golden Girls, window-shopping, or just smelling the roses. I've been back to the Island's annual rose show every year since that first time in 1993.

Second, I have become something of an activist, in my own way, deeply committed to helping newly-diagnosed women deal with their breast cancer more easily than I did.

I have initiated a programme in the surgical unit of the hospital, making relaxation tapes available to women before surgery. I obtained financing for the tapes from the Canadian Cancer Society, and I approached local businesses to donate portable cassette players and headsets. We now have enough replacement ear foams to last us through the next generation of Island women. God forbid they should ever need them.

For the past three years I have been a member of the Well Cells, a group of cancer survivors who hold various fundraisers. We once participated in a twenty-four-hour relay, and last year raised almost $9,000 through pledges, raffles, car washes, and the like. It is a very uplifting group, and we always have a good time.

I was also actively involved in the effort to make the core biopsy procedure available on the Island. It required the resources of a lot of groups and individuals, but the effort was worthwhile, and the equipment is now in operation and completely paid for. I am now self-taught in networking, fundraising and lobbying. What a change of pace for me!

It is interesting that in the process of helping others, I discover new things about myself every day. I live, I learn, and I grow. Suffice it to say, I have found my niche in life and consider myself blessed by the exhilarating feeling that comes from contributing to humanity. Being told that I am making a difference is the most distinguished badge I could ever hope to wear.

CAROLYN VANBUSKIRK

St. John, New Brunswick
Date of birth: May 25, 1943
Date of diagnosis: May 1988

When I finished reading Dr. Bernie Siegel's *Love, Medicine and Miracles*, an eerie feeling came over me. There I was on every page, my innermost thoughts and feelings, my actions and the specific way I conducted myself described in perfect detail. The book turned out to be my post-breast-cancer life's defining moment, when everything suddenly fell into place and I was liberated by awareness. Finally I had some reasons for my disease.

It took little effort to recognize myself in the portrait of the typical cancer patient. Like many women, I had been a nurturer and a caregiver throughout my life, unfailingly devoted to the happiness and welfare of others. I say this not out of regret, for I am proud of the path I have chosen and the moral code that has guided my life. I am a nurturer, always was and always will be. If I take issue with anything in my past, it's that I never acknowledged the need for clearing internal space for myself. And my breast cancer experience has taught me that I must. This is hard to remember, and even when remembered, it is often hard to do.

***

I was barely twenty-one and already married to Cecil for two years when I gave birth to our first son, Chris. Chris was a healthy, happy baby, and I was immediately overcome by the poetic romanticism of the times, anticipating in earnest the magical mystery tour of life. I felt much more than joy; I was in perfect harmony with the world. I understood God's design for humanity and the role I was to play in it. The Christmas of 1964, our first as a family, was the stuff of story-books and fairy tales, where everyone lives happily ever after. All my childhood dreams had come to pass.

This pristine optimism continued for three years. I had a wonderful husband, another baby on the way, and I had begun the career I always wanted, working in radio and writing for the newspaper. Then, suddenly, the clock struck twelve and my innocence was spent.

Our second son, Kelly, entered this world a very sick child. He was born with a congenital heart defect, and although we were told that surgery was a real option, we felt that the more time we could buy, the better. So we waited for him to get stronger, taking it one day at a time, living from moment to moment, emergency to emergency. The best and nearest specialists were in Halifax, and we drove the ten-hour return trip more often than I can recall, always at the mercy of our Maritime weather. Sometimes Kelly would be hospitalized. Other times there was nothing the doctors could do, and we were told to go home and keep a watchful eye on him.

Naturally, this ailing, frail child required a great deal of attention. I was fortunate to have a capable and loving aunt who was willing to help out, which enabled me to keep my job. On the days Auntie came over, I went to the office, working at home the rest of the week. It was an ad-lib kind of life, made ever more unsettling by Kelly's deteriorating health. By his fifth birthday, in addition to his heart condition, Kelly had gone totally deaf. Meanwhile, Chris was in his formative years and needed his mother just as much. I had, as they say, a lot of balls in the air.

I "busied" myself out of my anxieties by continuously over-committing. I was always on the go, fleeing from any situation that would leave me idle and permit me to think. But there is one recurring intermission in life that provides no dispensation. It is that sacredly intimate time in the stillness and the dark, between wakefulness and the onset of sleep, where thoughts roam like free radicals and nightmares are replayed, over and over, as if someone were playing with the remote control of our fears.

From the time of Kelly's birth, I had relied on prayer and the will of the Lord to sustain me. Ultimately, though, during a particularly exhausting vigil by Kelly's bed, I succumbed to the weight of my circumstance, and everything that was wrong with the world exploded around me. As I tended to my wounded spirit, I embraced my only recourse. I made a bargain with God. My part of the deal came to mind instantly. "If You heal my sick little boy," I told the Lord, "I will take a child no one wants and raise that child as my own."

Perhaps I was too naive.

Kelly was seven when we put our names on the adoption list. And since we had raised two babies of our own, we thought it would only be fair to ask for an older child. We didn't realize we were in the minority, that the demand for children — unlike the demand for babies — was limited. So, before long, I was dispatched to an emergency foster home to pick up Mary-Jane. She was exactly two years and one week old. The woman who came to the door didn't bother to hide her relief when she realized who I was. She shook her head in exasperation. "Thank God you got here," she exhaled, "before I killed her." My head spun with anger and confusion. What kind of surrogate was this who could speak about an innocent child this way?

Mary-Jane was in a playpen in the living room, and it was her eyes I first noticed. She was rolling them back in her head, as if she were having a seizure. She had the face of an untamed yearling, with those wild eyes and clenched teeth, her head shaking and jerking incessantly, as she tried to free herself from distress. Fragile, little hands squeezed the sides of the playpen, rattling it with a force much greater than I had ever seen from a two-year-old. The outline of her bones was visible through her jumper, a pronounced sign of malnutrition. And although we had been told that Mary-Jane was a "deprived" child, a momentary panic came over me when I realized the extent of her damage. But I simply let it pass. Mary-Jane was God's choice, not mine.

I left the emergency foster home with two small paper bags — one containing her clothes, the other her toys.

Even as we headed home, Mary-Jane began to exhibit the savage behaviour that would last the greater part of the next twelve years. Because she was unable to speak, she communicated with her body, flapping her arms, kicking her feet, pushing against the belt of her car seat with all her might. When we arrived at the house, she tore into my face and clawed at my eyes as I carried her from the car. I was the enemy. I was a grown-up.

Taking her across the threshold was an act that would permanently change my life, my husband's life, and our life as a family.

Once she was safe in her crib, I had a moment to myself and began to pray. "Lord, we can work this out. Mary-Jane simply needs love and the best physical and emotional attention we can give her."

But good intentions were not enough. Mary-Jane was unyielding, and no amount of kindness could rescue her. Sitting in her highchair, she would throw her food indiscriminately, ignoring everyone and everything in her trajectory. She would kick holes in the walls, tear the wallpaper, pound the furniture with her fists, and when I'd approach to soothe her, she'd strike out like an alley cat. One night, she climbed out of her crib and wandered downstairs to the kitchen, where she lit all four burners on the stove and almost set the house on fire. From that point onward, until she was mature enough to understand the consequences of her actions, I slept on a floormat outside her room.

The first time we took Mary-Jane to our pediatrician, he decided to place her in the hospital for assessment. About a month later, we were advised that in addition to her psychological damage, her nervous system was impaired, and that instead of living in a normal family environment she would have to be institutionalized for the rest of her life. I wasn't surprised. By then, family services had given us full details of her "deprivation," and Mary-Jane's story was not unlike a cheap, made-for-television movie of the week. Apparently, the only abuse she had been spared was sexual.

Family services now felt duty-bound to give us another child. We held a family meeting — as was our custom for all important issues — and we decided to refuse the offer. Although we knew we were starting from below zero, Mary-Jane had no one in the world other than the four of us. We couldn't leave her fate to the whim of administrators and bureaucrats.

I thus confirmed my commitment both to the Lord and to Mary-Jane. Determined more than ever to help this child, I vowed to consider her my own little girl. I even contemplated changing her name to Megan Elizabeth — the names I would have chosen had I given birth to a daughter. But Mary-Jane was so troubled I was concerned about taking away the one constant she had had in her life. I decided to simply call her Mary.

As you can imagine, having Mary for a daughter was a labour-intensive responsibility. In the beginning, whenever she was calm enough to allow me near her, I jumped at the chance. There were so many things to catch up on, to make up for. I remember cutting out pictures from magazines, pictures of things she had never seen before that now excited her — a dog, a house, a doll, a horse. In this manner, I introduced the world to her.

However, we found that taking responsibility for a damaged child in-volved sacrifices beyond the energy required to raise her. Often chided for our folly, we chose to keep her terrible behaviour under wraps, voluntarily cutting ourselves off from our friends.

Mealtimes were the worst. She would eat only with her hands, and when she grew out of throwing her food, she started hoarding her meals in her bedroom. She had a biological compulsion to know that food was closeby, to be able to touch it with her hands should she wake up in the dark of night, hungry or not. Sometimes the stench of a week's worth of stale dinners permeated the house. Spaghetti, roast chicken, tuna casserole, pizza, salad, and Jell-o regularly decayed under her bed. How could I have entertained? For years, our social life was virtually nonexistent.

During puberty Mary became husky and wide-shouldered, and was encouraged by her large physiology to become abusive toward me. My husband was on the road most of the time, which gave her plenty of opportunity. That she didn't do her homework was perhaps not abnormal, although I had never experienced this with the boys. But her way of settling the issue was to throw her books at me. The situation was larger than I could handle, and I took her to psychiatrists, psychologists, and social workers — to anyone who might be in a position to help. If you've ever seen the Helen Keller story, just substitute Mary in the role.

In the meantime, I had two other children to care for, each of whom needed my attention in his own, personal way. However, things were made easier by Kelly's steadily improving health, and I regularly thanked the Lord for that. He was hospitalized for the last time in the sixth grade, and in the following year his ears were rebuilt, allowing him to regain almost one hundred percent of his hearing. Gradually the hole in his heart filled in, and by the time he entered high school, he had become a formidable presence on the rugby field.

***

Nineteen eighty-six was a very bad year, and the start of a three-year period filled with hardship and tragedy.

With the onset of spring, Mary became smitten with the fancy that she might have a wonderful birth-mother somewhere who was grieving her. I tried to get her help in tracing her biological mother, but she rejected it, and me as well. None of this was my business. She had to do it her way. For Mary, leaving home at fourteen was like going to the beach. An outing. I called family services and alerted the child protection agency, but in the end there was nothing I could do. I had invested twelve years of my life, and all for naught. I was heartbroken.

While still in the throes of my daughter's betrayal, I was faced with yet another crisis. My mother, who was my soul-mate and best friend, was diagnosed with terminal bowel cancer. After Mom took ill, I wanted Dad to move in with us, but our family doctor insisted against it. Dad was partially paralysed from a stroke, and my only option was to place him in a Veterans' hospital. When I wrote my signature on the admission papers I was so overcome with grief and guilt that my hands literally trembled. It was a very sad event.

Mom died on June 7, 1987, and suddenly, at age forty-three, I felt like an orphan. The purest form of love was gone from my life. So too were sincerity, unconditional acceptance, honesty, and courage. When a mother dies, all these things go with her, and your world is never again complete.

Still, there was more. A few months after Mom's passing, Dad was diagnosed with a rare form of cancer, which was spreading quickly. And I, for some time, had been feeling a painful ridge protruding from the upper part of my right breast. Even though I had always been told that cancer doesn't hurt, I became very anxious and went to see our family doctor. "Mom has just died," I said, "my daughter's left home, and I just found out that my father has cancer. I'm falling apart here." Then I explained why I was worried about my breast and that I wanted to have a mammogram.

"You're way too young at forty-four," the doctor replied. "It isn't necessary."

In hindsight, I'll give him some leeway because it was 1987, and considering the prevailing wisdom on mammography, perhaps his response was simply more conservative than ignorant. But in light of the ensuing events, I strongly resent his conduct.

After a few rounds of "are you sure it isn't necessary?" and "yes, I'm sure," I decided it was time to wrestle him to the floor. By then I was used to fighting. For Kelly, for Dad, and the Lord knows, for my mother. For the morphine shots that never arrived on time. For IVs to be reinserted, bedpans to be brought or removed, baths to be given, and for everything else that could legally be done to ease her pain.

Because I was not an emergency case, it took me three months to get a mammogram. Little did I know that I would soon find myself entering yet another unfamiliar and frightening dimension in my life's passage. I didn't know why God was testing me so.

***

In the winter of 1988 my preeminent concern was my father. He was undergoing standard cancer treatment — surgery followed by adjuvant therapy. The scene was ominously familiar. Dad was in the same hospital, on the same floor, just a few feet down the hall from where mother died, and where I had wept and slept and held her hand.

My time and energy were scarce. Not much remained after being with Dad, and of the little that was left my husband and two sons were the beneficiaries. By the end of each day I was running on empty. Perhaps once — maybe for an instant — I thought of following up on the results of my mammogram, but I shrugged it off as a waste of time. Everything was okay, I reasoned. Otherwise, someone would have called me.

I must have sleepwalked through that winter. I didn't remember a single blizzard. Suddenly it was unusually bright in the morning, and Mary, I realized, had already turned sixteen!

I was on my way to visit Dad one morning, managing little more than a peek at our blossoming yellow tulips, when I remembered that I needed to renew an antibiotic prescription. I raced toward the doctor's office, planning a quick entrance and exit, but I was stopped dead in my tracks. "Before I write the prescription," the doctor said, "we'd better talk about your mammogram." He asked me to sit down.

The next thing I knew he was speaking in esoteric cancer language, using words such as calcification, biopsy, and lesion. Instantly my mind scrambled for a safe corner. "How is your new baby daughter?" I asked, and "Do you think you'll be moving to a bigger house now?" This ridiculous banality was the good little girl in me talking, the socially polite, well-bred, "put your best foot forward and not in your mouth" debutante. I should have shaken him in his shoes and screamed, "Where have you been for the last three months! Why didn't you call me? Why didn't anybody call me?"

I left his office with a referral for a surgeon and my radiology report. As I headed toward my car, I noticed several benches on the grass bordering the parking lot. They were very alluring, with backs of intricate wrought-iron curlicues and legs shaped in delicate Queen Anne style. I slowed my gait and staked out my territory, walking toward the bench farthest from parked cars and perambulating humans. The referral slip was still in my hands, and I stared at it, examining the name, searching for clues to the man who would play God with my life. Then I reread the radiology report. I had two lesions, one with tentacles — or whatever the appropriate medical term is — the other without.

When I called the surgeon's office for an appointment, the receptionist found it hard to believe that I had gone uninformed about a highly suspicious mammogram for three months, then blithely booked me with a two-and-a-half-week delay. After my pleading and cajoling and whatever else I could think of, she relented. I got an appointment two days hence.

It was a late May afternoon, and the surgeon's waiting room was packed. I sat for hours, flipping through magazines, looking at the women who went in and came out of the examination room, staring at their chests through my dark sunglasses, trying to ascertain who had only one breast, who had none. By the time my turn arrived, it was seven o'clock. The only thing that kept me sane was the anticipation of imminent relief. I expected to be reassured by the calm, comforting wisdom of a sage who had seen hundreds of cases like mine, hundreds of false alarms. Instead, I met an irritable self-proclaimed saviour, as stingy with his words as with his manners. Of the two suspicious lesions, he believed one to be a benign cyst. Without further adieu, he inserted a needle into my breast, drew out some fluid, raised it to eye-level for both of us to see — "See?" — and then flushed it down the sink. There was no explanation. I sat motionless, watching in shock as part of my body slid down the drainpipe like the dregs of a day-old cup of coffee.

As for the second suspicious lesion, the one with the "tentacles," the surgeon recommended that "we" watch it. He told me to return in three months. I drove home physically numb and emotionally drained, having recently watched cancer take a lethal foothold on both my parents. Was *I* going to sit back and be swallowed up too?

The following morning I tore through the streets of the town, aiming for my family doctor's office. I firmly presented him with two requests. First, I wanted another mammogram. Immediately. Second, I wanted a list of every breast surgeon in the city. I had too much experience with cancer to know that "watching" it was not what I needed. I needed a biopsy, and I would knock on every door until I found a surgeon willing to do it.

From there, events proceeded rather quickly. Armed with my second mammogram and my blackmail list, I beat a path back to the surgeon's door. I was in no mood to beg for help, and I had no patience for shoulder-shrugs and nebulous answers. This time, however, there was no hesitation. The surgeon would perform the biopsy at the first available opportunity. Maybe the next day. At most I would have to wait two.

I took a detour on the way home. It was a case of now or never, not a minute to spare. I arrived in a complete frenzy, but I made it. The store was still open, thank goodness.

I had spent forty-five years on this planet as a female and had never owned a pullover. I was not the sweater type, I guess. In fact, I don't remember borrowing any from friends when we did that adolescent girlish thing of exchanging clothes. I had never worn one for going to the market, for building snowmen in the yard, or for playing golf on a cool, autumn afternoon. Well, my dear, I thought to myself, tonight may be your last chance. You may have only a few hours left with two breasts, so you'd better show off what you have while you still have it, even if you're no competition for Pamela Lee.

I have never been a big spender, but this purchase was different. Much to the delight of the salesclerk, I declared, "Money's no object." To this day, Cecil doesn't know how much I paid for that crayola-indigo cashmere turtleneck, imported from Scotland.

The salesclerk was about to place it in a box when I stopped her. "I'd like to put it on," I said, and disappeared into the dressing room, asking her to pack, instead, the silk blouse I had worn that day. She was still manipulating the proper fold for the lace that adorned it, when I emerged in all my resonant splendour. Expressionless, she said, "You know, I have several pairs of pants that would look *very smart* with that sweater."

"Well, yes," I replied, "some are wise, and some are otherwise." I was quoting the last line of the newspaper column I had written the night before, some old proverb. My only other choice would have been to tell her the story of my life. Later, when I thought about my behaviour (or was it arrogance?), I realized it was not me, but rather the threat of breast cancer talking. Spontaneous spunk. Militant moxy. There are no rules when your life is under siege.

At home I changed into a skirt that matched my sweater reasonably well, and decided I was rather pleased with my looks. But it was too little, too late, and I quickly turned to more important things — the daunting task of reassuring my family. I had always been strong, independent, and able to take care of myself, which meant that I could pull this off as long as I remained in character. "A biopsy is really no big deal," I began, "I'll be just fine. Besides, the whole thing is probably a huge mistake. Seems you just can't get good help these days, ha-ha." But the more I tried, the quieter my husband became, and that scared me. Cecil is usually very optimistic.

After dinner I started to prepare the house for my absence. I cleaned, did the laundry, baked some cookies, and cooked a few meals to throw in the freezer. In the midst of this activity, the phone rang, and I was told to check into the hospital by ten a.m. the next day. "I'll give you a ride on my way to rugby practice," Kelly volunteered, nonchalantly.

When we retired for the night, I took off my sweater and placed it on the cedar chest at the foot of our bed, directly in my line of vision. I wanted to be able to see it should I wake in the middle of the night. However, that didn't happen because I never went to sleep. I had spent many, many sleepless nights before, first agonizing over Kelly, then Mary, then Mom and Dad. This time it was my turn. Oddly, the fear wasn't any deeper — it was just different. Death didn't scare me, for I knew I would be going to a beautiful place, but I was terrified by the process of dying.

Kelly dropped me off at the hospital entrance, and I went to the admissions office alone, the way I had planned. Registration didn't take very long, and I soon found myself on the surgical floor looking at familiar faces. "Who is it this time, Carolyn?" they asked. When I gave them my answer, there was a stunned silence. Even the nurses with whom I had argued over my parents' care reached out with reassuring hugs. But the expression of pity on their faces only bolstered my determination. I have since realized that the most difficult thing to accept about pity is the likelihood that you have earned it.

At some point between the pre-op tests and an exhausting procedure known as a needle localization, the surgeon made his obligatory appearance. I didn't care about the details, I told him. There was only one issue I wanted to discuss. Did he think I would need a mastectomy? "Your family history scares me," he replied. Then his beeper went off and he left.

When it was all over and I was back in my bed, groggy from the anaesthetic and only half-awake, I saw my family gathered together. They didn't have to say anything. I knew by their presence that I had cancer.

Beholden to the makers of demerol, I closed my eyes and allowed a numbing void to envelop my body before slipping into blissful oblivion for the night.

Morning was a different story. The bandages were wrapped tightly around my chest and back, and I could neither feel nor see what was beneath them. But I clearly remembered what the surgeon had said when I was still in the recovery room. He had saved my breast — or fifty-five percent of it — and now I felt curiously ungrateful for that. I knew this disease. I held great respect for cancer and I didn't want to leave anything to chance. Rather my breast than my life.

Over the next several days, as I waited for the diagnostics that would determine my chances of survival, my nerves were put to the test. And I earned high marks, falling apart bit by bit, cell by cell, with each passing hour. Yes, I thought of making another bargain with God, but I readily dismissed it. I had made the first one for my son, and in my mind it had been for life. I would never do anything to jeopardize that. Instead, I prayed. "Well, Lord, I did the best I could. Let the chips fall where they may, Amen. Thy will be done." This was good enough for me.

Finally, all my test results were in, and they were consistent. The cancer hadn't spread. In light of such good news my confidence returned, and I thought that perhaps the surgical procedure had been appropriate after all. Now all I needed was twenty sessions of radiation and I could put this whole sordid episode behind me. Whew. Let's go home.

***

Just when I was getting used to the idea that I could keep my breasts *and* my life, the curtain rose on act two.

The scene: my first appointment with the radiation oncologist. Clutching my file in her hands, she stared at me and asked point-blank, "Are you satisfied with your surgery?"

"*Satisfied?*" I asked, incredulously. What did she mean was I satisfied? What kind of question was that!

I don't know if she impressed me because she was a woman — and could imagine what it must be like to sacrifice a breast — or because she was the first medical professional who appeared to show a genuine interest in me.

"In your case, no amount of radiation is going to kill the rest of the cancer," she began. "You should have had a mastectomy."

She went on to explain her diagnosis and urged me to contact my surgeon. She told me to insist that he remove the remainder of my breast. But I was tired. I had reached the end of my rope. I had fought for a mammogram, to see a surgeon, to have a biopsy. There had been too much confrontation in my life and I didn't have any fight left in me.

Thank the Lord that the oncologist valued my life more than a politics, for the next thing I knew my husband and I were summoned to a conference convened, no doubt, at her request. There were several attending physicians present, but my surgeon was conspicuously absent. We were told "officially" that a mastectomy would be more effective than radiation. What did I think?

What did I think? Lots of things. I thought there was a prescribed procedure for breast cancer surgery. I thought that doctors would take care of me. That they knew what they were doing. That's what I thought. I was unprepared for this type of personal involvement in my disease. I didn't know that there was so much controversy over treatment. I didn't know that women were expected to make life-saving decisions for themselves, by themselves.

Losing the remaining fifty-five percent of a dangling breast — which was not much to speak of in the first place — was a small price to pay for my life. "Let's go with the mastectomy," I replied.

My tone had a familiar ring to it. An order from a boss, an instruction from a coach, a military mission? "Let's go with a mastectomy." In other words, "let's do it!" How utterly bizarre. When I wasn't looking, the world had turned upside down.

***

I love going to auctions. That was where the hospital found me when I was summoned for my stand-by mastectomy.

It was just outside the operating room that my surgeon, fully gowned and masked, mumbled some semblance of an apology. I readily accepted. I was prepped and strapped to a gurney. It was he who held the knife.

Oddly, the surgery itself was almost anticlimactic. I was an old hand at this and knew every step in the process: the anaesthesia, the bandages, the drainage tubes and the mandatory arm exercises.

One afternoon an auburn-haired, well-dressed, healthy-looking woman knocked on my door. She was a volunteer with Reach to Recovery, and had had a mastectomy herself. I beamed when she told me that she was a ten-year survivor. Wow! I had read about these women, such as Nancy Reagan, but I didn't know any breast cancer survivors personally. Now, here she was, a living testament to hope. What I remember best about her are the words that eventually became my credo. She was the first to say to me, "Start by being good to Carolyn, and the rest will take care of itself."

On my first day home, after everyone had left for the day, the dam finally broke. Despair gushed from every pressurized pore, like water from an open hydrant; even the rafters shook. I howled like this for weeks, until the backlog of tears had cleared. In the evening, however, I donned my stoic wardrobe and slipped into character, trying very hard to re-establish an orderly routine. "Don't worry about me. I'm fine," I insisted. I am their mother and wife, *of course* I didn't want them to worry about me. And I did feel fine, *under the circumstances.*

These initial few weeks, perhaps even months, were emotionally the most difficult. There were no more doctors, nurses, or other health professionals buzzing efficiently about. There were no more tears from my family. The attention was gone. I had survived the crisis. Now what? The world, I discovered, is made up of only two kinds of women. Those who have breast cancer and those who don't.

At home, no one wanted to talk about the ordeal. After all, I showed no signs of illness. I required neither radiation nor chemotherapy. I wasn't bald and I didn't throw up. As far as my family was concerned, life had returned to normal. Their wife and mother was back, exactly the way she had been before she left. And that was how they behaved.

One evening, soon after the total mastectomy, my elder son asked if I would make a little dinner party for him and a friend.

This was when it hit me. I was running a fever and was sick to my stomach from a lingering infection. *I was recovering from breast cancer!* Life was *not* the way it used to be. *I* was not the way I used to be. And although I rejected any form of pity or sympathy, I felt totally helpless and misunderstood. I wanted my family to recognize, not ignore, that I was weaker than a kitten and unable to perform as usual. Pretending that my breast cancer had never happened didn't make me feel better. It only made *them* feel better.

"If you want a dinner party, you're most welcome to have one," I told Chris. "The food is in the fridge, but you will have to prepare it." Chris looked at me with alarm. This wasn't the gung-ho mother he knew and loved. Why was I behaving like this? Moms are not allowed to be sick. Neither are wives.

A few weeks after my homecoming, my husband and I went out to dinner with another couple. I was rubbery-legged and queasy but agreed to go. When the woman lit her tenth cigarette of the evening, I told Cecil I wanted to go home. Cecil, on the other hand, was having a good time, and took me aside where he bawled me out, ending with something to the effect that, "You're okay now. You're very lucky. So what's the problem?"

At that moment I didn't feel like being told how lucky I was. We went home and had a huge row. It felt good to let the anger out.

There were other times like this. I remember Cecil saying, "So, you're a bit wounded. Now get on with it." But his hurtful words and actions were not born of malice; I knew that. They were reflections of his point of view, his desires, and his needs. Not mine. He didn't know about how I got out of bed at night, after he fell asleep, and lay awake on the couch with my thoughts. He didn't know that I felt like an old woman, that I questioned my sexual identity, that I wondered if his staying with me wasn't simply his way of making the best of a bad situation. And how could he know about the recurring nightmares — or the nightmares about recurrence — the fear of dying, the images of IVs and breathing machines hooked into my body.

I missed my mother terribly. She would have been able to help and comfort me. She would have said, "You know, Carolyn, it's enough that you are just living and breathing. And I think you are wonderful." Sometimes, in the middle of the night, when I'm awake and the house is still, I am sure I hear her whispering to me.

My emotional convalescence took about six months. After I had spent all my tears of anger and anguish, it was time to get myself together.

I had been on staff at the *Saint John Telegraph Journal* for some time, and was still a regular contributor when I decided to go public with my story. Journalism may be my profession, but this time it would also double as therapy. I must add that I had never been a public person. I used to be so Victorian, in fact, that I had trouble ordering chicken breasts at the butcher shop.

The paper devoted the entire front page of its Saturday "People" section to me, including a large picture taken shortly after my surgery, when I had gathered the clan together and commandeered a family portrait. I was wearing an ivory silk and lace dress, a gift from my mother before she died. I had been saving it secretly for my funeral, but in one sporadic moment of vanity, I ditched that idea and donned it for the photograph.

The story ran on February 4, 1989, and the reaction to it was, as my grandson would say, "awesome." It tied up all the mammogram machines in the city for weeks. The phone rang off the wall. Newly diagnosed women were calling for advice, as were cancer support groups and other organizations. I had found my voice in advocacy.

Breast cancer has always been talked about in hushed tones, and this is partly our fault. Women have been quiet about it for too long. Even ten years after the fact, I am still angry about the way I was ignored and told to go away. If I hadn't insisted on a mammogram, I would be history by now.

What's the big secret here? Breast cancer has been around since the days of our great grandmothers. Women need to know the facts. They must learn to be responsible for their own health, their own bodies. So I shouted, "Listen up! There's something you must know. I have a big secret! I have breast cancer. And one out of nine women will get it in her lifetime. You could be next. Now let's go out and do something about it."

Breast cancer is not the best thing that has ever happened to me, but it has given me the freedom to pursue what I want to pursue, and to live my life the way I want. I now give myself permission to sit down and read two chapters of a book. I've lost all interest in housework. If the house gets messy, I'll spiff it up enough to make it presentable. Big deal. And it's the same with cooking. I've learned that frozen food is not lethal.

I value my independence. I don't need a title and a business card to define who I am. I know who I am. My disease gave me a crash course in self-reflection.

I have also changed my attitude toward money. Now I go on little spending sprees. Silly stuff for the grandchildren. It's my way of saying, "Hey, I'm happy to be alive." And, "Hey, I'm not leaving it for the next wife!"

Afterword

I would be remiss if I left you with the wrong impression. In fact, there is a happy ending to my story, at least up to this point in my life.

I'll begin with myself. After the mastectomy in May 1988, I had a lot of trouble with my other breast. It had always been fibrocystic, and although subsequent mammograms didn't show anything specific, my breast contained many palpable masses. This time the doctors were more cautious and more suspicious, and it was suggested I have a second mastectomy. I waited a year to regain my physical strength before I went ahead with it. As it turned out, the doctors were right. Pre-cancerous cells were hiding everywhere, mostly behind the benign tumours. To tell you the truth, having my other breast removed didn't bother me at all. If anything, I am more balanced. People tell me I carry myself better now. And besides, I felt so stupid with one breast just dangling there.

As for Cecil, somewhere along the way he seems to have made a hundred-and-eighty-degree turn. Three years ago, I was asked to speak to a group of nursing students about caring for patients with cancer. But I had been suffering from the flu the day before and didn't want to go. When I mentioned to Cecil how badly I felt about reneging, he asked, "Would you feel any better if I went in your place?" I had no idea what he had in mind. "If *you* went?" I questioned. "Yes," he answered, "I'm as much an expert as you on the subject. I'm the one who made all the mistakes."

After it was over, I was told that my husband brought the house down. Everyone fell in love with him. By the end of his speech there wasn't a dry eye in the place.

I still have a habit of over-committing, but now Cecil is always there to nag, "Where is my freedom girl?" And then I remember the Reach to Recovery volunteer who told me to be good to Carolyn. To make room for myself.

Chris, my elder son, became an Anglican priest and has a parish within a three-hour drive from here, weather permitting. He and his wife have three children — Kelly, Isabelle and Gregory. When Chris told me that they had chosen my mother's name for their only daughter, I'm sure you can imagine how moved I was. And I knew my mother was smiling in heaven.

My own Kelly overcame his serious illness to play on Canada's official rugby team when he was younger. Now he's a handsome, married, thirty-year-old lawyer who still calls me every night.

Last, but not least, is Mary. She located her mother in a bar, "drunk as a skunk," and was rejected by her again. It was a sorrowful episode in her life, but Mary eventually came to terms with it. And she also came to terms with her growing-up years, including her attitude toward me. In 1990, four years after she left, she came home and got married. She has turned into a wonderful young woman and is an exceptional mother. She named her son Steven Christopher, his middle name after her brother. And, in spite of all predictions to the contrary, she leads a very normal life.

Mary loves to come home and visit with me — away from the pollution and the noise of the city. In the summer, she and little Steven vacation here, and I revel in the chance to be a full-time grandmother. What joy!

Gert Batist

Montreal, Quebec
Date of birth: October 14, 1927
Date of diagnosis: October 1973

It was the fall of 1973, just before the High Holidays — a most special time of the year for me. I grew up in an Orthodox Jewish home, and the first ten days of the New Year always meant more to me than simply going to *shul*, showing off my new outfit to anyone who would acknowledge my presence, sticking my nose up at the boys, or hanging on to my mother's skirt listening to the latest gossip, though all of this was fun, especially the gossip. I may not have known the people being talked about, but that didn't matter. I liked to act grown-up and pretend to understand the deep significance of the ladies' observations, insightful commentaries, and acute fashion critiques.

No, the High Holidays also meant joy of family and celebrations. I can remember as a young child sitting at our huge dining room table on Rosh Hashanah, as overwhelmed by the quantity of food laid out in front of me (which I could never reach and was too shy to ask for) as by the number of people around me — my *bubby* and *zaidie*, aunts and uncles, first and second cousins, newcomers by marriage, and before I knew it, competition: brand-new babies. I was convinced that everyone in the world was related to me.

When I was eleven, my mother gave birth to twins — a boy and a girl — and her health began to deteriorate. She needed a trainable apprentice and, being the eldest, I inherited a major role in our family life at a rather young age. In our culture it is the responsibility — indeed the privilege — of the women of the house to create a home that exudes a beautiful way of life, observing traditions and preparing elaborate, special meals of fantastic quantities for all the various festivals and holidays.

These childhood experiences stayed with me throughout my life, and when I became the so-called matriarch of my own family, the High Holidays, in particular, inspired me to flavour the household with a solemn sense of togetherness and family harmony.

By the time 1973 rolled around, my husband and I had been married for twenty-six years and had four children — girl, boy, girl, boy. (I credit him for that. He is very organized.) The two eldest were not living with us anymore. One daughter had recently graduated and was on her own — after all, it *was* the seventies — and one son was a first-year medical student at McGill University. I was anxious to have everyone home, together again. Anticipating the presence of both my husband's and my own extended families, the idea of preparing for the holidays filled me with excitement and a little trepidation; it would be a lot of work. But I did it with devotion. Well, all right, at times it seemed as if I were catering a *simcha* we were so many, thank God. And today, we still are. Twenty-five of us: children, grand-children, Phil and me.

The only doctor I saw on a regular basis was my gynaecologist, and because of the hectic two weeks that lay ahead of me, I always scheduled my annual check-up prior to the holidays. I wanted it out of the way, so that I could concentrate on only those obligations that concerned family.

By and large everything was fine that year, but my gynaecologist thought he detected a lump attached to my breast bone. He couldn't really be sure, so he wanted me to see a breast man. I remember chewing gum as I entered the doctor's office, something that was considered quite rude in those days, but I didn't care. I was nervous. After Dr. M. examined me, he said, "You can stop chewing your gum now, Mrs. Batist. It's nothing."

Phew, I thought to myself. Then, in an instant, he undermined my sense of relief, explaining that he still wanted to send me for a mammogram. Twenty-five years ago, there was no such thing as routine screening, and a woman went for a mammogram only if her doctor had found something suspicious.

Dr. M. didn't have the guts to call me with the results, perhaps because doctors "didn't make mistakes" back then. They were not viewed as ordinary people, and thus they couldn't have ordinary faults. And in 1973 cancer was not an appropriate topic of discussion, even between doctors and patients. Dr. M. decided instead to call my husband at the office, relying on him to break the news to me.

My husband was not well equipped to be the first to learn about my illness. Not that we didn't have a solid marriage — we celebrated our golden wedding anniversary in 1996. But Phil was old-fashioned. He saw himself as the sole provider, while I was the homemaker and caregiver, whose primary responsibility entailed raising our four children. With such a traditional division of labour in our family, serious illnesses could not be accommodated. Sore throats, earaches and chicken pox, yes. But certainly nothing "grown-up." So on the day that Dr. M. called, my husband's world collapsed.

I was no hero either. This could not be happening to me, I bemoaned. I am not ready to die. I am forty-six years old, and my youngest is only thirteen. He had just been *Bar Mitzvahed*. What will happen to my children? How will my husband survive?

And the timing! It couldn't have been worse. In the intervening years, I've discovered that one of the great mysteries of life is that a breast cancer diagnosis always appears at the most inopportune hour. Or is it just that we don't appreciate the splendour of our lives' rhythms until we are stopped dead in our tracks?

That evening, Phil and I hid ourselves from the children, bereft, as if we were sitting *shiva*. Among his many qualities, Phil, thank God, is a fighter, a very strong personality who has never allowed himself to be defeated by circumstance. He likes to be in control, and he is not one to be daunted by new, even scary, situations. True to form, after a brief period of premature mourning, he quickly regained his composure and went into action, determined to find me the best cancer surgeon in the city. In less than a day, we had a name.

When Phil and I talked it over, however, we decided to put off seeing Dr. P. until after the holidays. Actually, this was more my decision than his, even though I knew that I'd need every ounce of my willpower to hide my emotions from the family. I was scared and very, very angry. My father, you see, had had tuberculosis when I was a child, and my mother had been so worried about it, that she had taken me for X-rays every week. Meanwhile, my husband was a heavy smoker, and no matter what I tried with him — admonishment or pleas — nothing worked. Our house was always full of smoke. As for me, two years before my cancer diagnosis, when I went to give blood, I learned that I was anaemic and was advised to see a doctor. But I just hadn't bothered. So there you have it. Three very good reasons for my illness. And I didn't know who was more to blame — my mother, my husband, or myself.

Gradually, however, as the High Holidays approached, my anger gave way to self-reflection. This period in the Jewish calendar is the holiest, requiring that every Jew examine herself in all aspects of her life — all deeds, actions, thoughts — and I had always taken the spiritual aspect of the holidays very seriously. From birth, part of me has been defined by my religion, just as part of me, from the age of forty-six, will forever be defined by breast cancer.

According to Judaism, everything that we do, or say, or think becomes a matter of permanent record. On the first day of the New Year — Rosh Hashanah — also known as the Day of Judgement, Jewish tradition tells us that God sits enthroned in a hall of justice. The books, in which all the deeds of humankind are inscribed, lie in front of Him, and He pronounces judgement on all creatures of the earth. On the tenth day — Yom Kippur — this judgement is sealed. In between, during the ten days of penitence, we can ask for the forgiveness of our sins through specific activities such as prayer, charity, and good deeds.

Reflecting on my circumstances, I couldn't help but question whether I had brought this illness on myself. What terrible things had I done to deserve this? Had I crossed the line, or hurt anyone? Had I allowed bad thoughts to enter my mind? Was this a form of payment or punishment?

Then the Yom Kippur war broke out, with the Arabs invading Israel at night while everyone was at prayer. I have family there. I don't think there is a single Jew alive who doesn't have relations of one sort or another in Israel. When I was eighteen, I remember nervously listening to the radio broadcast of the United Nations' vote on the creation of a Jewish state. Later, I made frequent trips to Israel and worked for various North American charities, mostly raising money for Israel's development. As my country, Canada is in my heart; but as my heritage, Israel is in my soul. At the core of my existence, I thought both Israel and I were fighting for our lives, and when Israel won, my own determination was bolstered.

So, as I was whipping up my matzo ball mixture (you should *always* whip the egg whites), contemplating the meaning of my life, and seeking an understanding with God, I realized that the opportunity to influence my destiny lay within my grasp. I could not change the fact that I had breast cancer. This was the way life was supposed to be for me. But I could change my fate. I stopped focusing on the why part of it and, instead, began to think about *how* I was now going to proceed. I concluded that this had happened to me for a reason, and resolved to turn my experience into a positive one.

By the grace of the powers around me, the holidays passed without incident, and on the twelfth day of *Tishrei,* Phil and I went to see the surgeon.

Dr. P. was a highly respected physician with a reputation for performing only radical mastectomies, even though proponents of the modified Halsted procedure were already emerging in the late seventies. I was told that this was his preferred method and that a radical mastectomy was the type of operation I would likely undergo if he were to become my surgeon. With Dr. P. it wasn't a matter of choice. He maintained that the only way to save a woman's life was by removing the entire breast and everything in its vicinity. And everyone maintained that Dr. P. was the best.

When I first met him, he spoke and I listened. His speech was laconic; there wasn't much discussion. Most of our conversation concerned procedure, and I learned that the first test I would have to undergo was a thermogram, which had been scheduled for the following day.

And so the fact of losing my breast, all the lymph nodes under my arm, and my chest muscles on the entire upper-left side of my body was settled in a matter of minutes, and that is simply the way life was back then.

That I would become so utterly deformed was a devastating revelation. During the previous three weeks, I had struggled only with a notion. In Dr. P.'s office that notion became a horrific reality. I witnessed the disintegration of my resolve as surely as if I had been in the war, hit by a bomb. And I left his office in a daze, quite certain I would wake up and discover that this was happening to someone else.

It had taken a long time and a great deal of effort for me to come this far in life. Breast cancer was not part of my plans.

***

In spite of my traditional, Orthodox upbringing, I had always been individualistic, with strong views and a unique sense of myself. However, finding the balance between the fulfilment of my own desires and those of the influential others in my life had long been a struggle. And, as with all compromises, one side usually received priority over the other. Just to give you one example, as a young girl I decided that when I got married, I would have lots and lots of children — seven, eight, nine, ten, I had no specific number in mind. But some people with whom I was close influenced me otherwise. "Why on earth would you want to do that? In this day and age?" they asked. "Because children make your life rich, more complete," I replied, and even though that was how I felt, in the end I acquiesced and settled for four.

As for work, I had always wanted to have just a little part-time job to prove to myself that I was talented and capable of earning money. Today we would probably refer to this as an issue of self-esteem. So I became a real-estate agent, but with a twist. I would spend my days in the office reviewing all the old, unsold files that had been more-or-less written off. Then I would examine the current list of clients who hadn't yet purchased, and match up the two. It was a simple approach but successful, and I derived a great deal of satisfaction from my ingenuity, not to mention my commissions. Unfortunately, my husband preferred that I stop. So I did.

I soon found myself a more "suitable" interest and for many years became involved in community service as an active participant with charitable organizations. There came a time, however, when this type of work could no longer provide me with intellectual satisfaction, and because I had never had the opportunity to finish high school, I felt something was missing from my life. This motivated me to take an adult education course. Just one course. Then one course led to another, and another, and I quickly found my studies taking a more serious turn. Eventually I decided to enrol in the Thomas More Institute for Adult Education, which would later allow me to pursue university studies.

Just as an aside, there was a very interesting question on my final exam for the English essay course. It was: "What would you prefer, shame or guilt?" When I read it, I had to pinch myself and could hardly contain my laughter. I almost felt as if I were cheating. Guilt? Who in their right mind would want me — a Jewish mother — to write about guilt? For marks, no less! It was too good to be true. Suffice it to say, I aced the exam.

My pre-university studies lasted a couple of years, long enough for everyone to get used to the idea that I wanted to keep going. I was finally doing something that was important to me. When I entered the sociology programme at Concordia University, I was forty-four years old. I can recall vividly the first day of classes. I was the only adult enrolled in daytime studies and hadn't realized how many problems I would face. Where do I sit? What do I do with my purse? When do I go to the bathroom? Where *is* the bathroom? How do I address the professors, some of whom could easily be my own children? Hundreds of seemingly trivial tasks became issues of utmost importance. The molehill *was* a mountain because in that environment, on the first day of school, I felt like a mole. But just for a day. By the second day, everything was a breeze.

And then, two years into my studies, came breast cancer.

In 1973, the world was not a pleasant place if one received a cancer diagnosis. Instead of sympathy, a woman encountered alienation. Instead of comfort, she received pity. Instead of encouragement, she was treated to silence. Reason bowed to emotion, as it so often does, and people were afraid to be around her for fear of catching this mysterious affliction. In everyone's mind, cancer was the exordium of death. Why? Because those who lived long lives after surviving cancer rarely told a soul, whereas everyone knew when someone died from it. It was a very lopsided situation.

The evening before my operation, the nurse preparing me for surgery just couldn't contain herself. "You know, Mrs. Batist, you're a very brave woman," she said. "You're not even crying. If this were happening to me, I'd throw myself out the window." Imagine! This was a medical professional talking. "In that case," I responded, "you should have your head examined." That shut her up, at least for the night.

My hospital stay lasted three weeks because my arm filled up with water, and they were afraid to release me. What a different environment we lived in at the time. If a person was sick, she was hospitalized. End of discussion. But that was only one side of the good old days. There was, of course, the other side — the one that attested to a certain societal immaturity, to a time of inadvertent prejudices and whispers, when some truths were ignorantly relegated to the status of shameful secrets, and patients, presumably for their own good, were protected from knowing their own fate. Not surprisingly, just two days after my surgery I couldn't contact Dr. P. I guess he didn't think it was necessary for me to see him. He had done his job. And then he left for vacation.

Even the results of my lymph node biopsy were given to me by an intern. I remember this young fellow coming into my room and saying, rather awkwardly, that he had some bad news to tell me. Then, noticing the name over my hospital bed, he suddenly became very agitated. Without moving his head, he shifted his eyes down toward the charts in his hands and realized that the two names didn't match. He had made a mistake. My lymph nodes were negative.

His attitude, however, was somewhat flippant. He said it was all a matter of luck, anyway. I could walk out on the street and get killed by a car. True. Or I could live to be one hundred and twenty — *bis* 120, as we say in Yiddish. Frankly, I agreed with him. I believe that we all have a destiny, but I also believe that there are things we can do to influence that destiny.

***

Those three weeks in the hospital gave me plenty of time to think.

I cannot remember how long it took, but once I began to see things logically, I didn't even have to decide. Even before I made the decision to change, I already had.

My life up to that point had been very much influenced by the significant others around me, so it was my duty to advise the most significant of these first — my husband and my mother. Shortly after coming home from the hospital, I pulled them each aside and announced, "I am a changed person now." My tone was serious, filled with determination. They both reacted in the same manner, sensing the gravity of the situation, and asked apprehensively, "Gert, what exactly does that mean?"

I replied, "It is quite simple, really. All my life everyone has felt that they had a right to interfere, to tell me what I should or should not do. And I allowed them. I gave in. Why? Because I wanted the world to love me. Well, not any more. From now on I have to love myself. I come first." Although I spoke in earnest, or perhaps because of it, these discussions were uncomfortable, and I felt I had to say something mitigating. It was not the most shining demonstration of my intellect. "Don't worry," I told them, "this doesn't mean that I am going to do terrible things from now on."

I tried to explain that coming first meant that I would live in the "now." That tomorrow would be today. Whatever it was I had to do, or wanted to do, I was going to do it today. I was going to celebrate every event, because life itself is a celebration.

Putting myself first also meant that I would go back to school, not because I wanted to earn my degree, but because I wanted to fill every day with learning. And shortly after being released from the hospital, I managed to attend even the first day of classes in the fall semester. I was still somewhat weak and self-conscious, but I was undeterred. (I graduated four years later, at the age of fifty, with a BA in sociology.)

Of course, it was somewhat of an exaggeration to use the words "putting myself first," and I didn't mean them literally. My religion had taught me that we are on this earth to serve others. But this does not imply that we should forsake ourselves in the bargain. And the three weeks I had spent in the hospital had opened up my mind to many possibilities.

First, I planned to become a Reach for Recovery volunteer. I had received a visit from one of these volunteers while in the hospital, and I will never forget how much better I felt afterwards. I, too, wanted to make a difference. I wanted to be the voice of reason and comfort amidst the prejudices and misunderstandings of a cancer diagnosis.

Allow me to recount just two brief incidents that reflect the mentality of the times. I once went to visit a patient whose relations had gathered at her bedside the day after her surgery. According to custom, I asked the family to step outside while I talked with her. I found her lying in her bed, despondent, eyes glazed, staring at nothing in particular. As a volunteer, this was not an unusual sight for me, but it was no less gut-wrenching. I was well trained, though, and knew what to say. "I know how you feel," I said. "It is terrible what has happened to you. Breast cancer was a terrible experience for me, too. And today I'm alive and healthy and happy. Don't worry, this too shall pass."

As I was about to leave the room, she whispered that she wanted me to be very careful with her family and never to use the "C-word" in their presence. Outside, I was pulled aside by a family member, and when we were a sufficient distance from the others, she said, almost reproachfully, "Whatever you talked about in there, I hope you didn't use that C-word with her." I lied, of course, because I didn't want to add to the burden this family had already taken upon itself.

Later, when I worked as a volunteer in radiotherapy, I came across many patients who were equally adamant about keeping their diagnosis a secret. They would lose their jobs, they said, their friends. One man, an accountant, was so scared of telling his boss that he decided to have prostate surgery during his vacation.

***

After breast cancer, life became a series of improvisations, as I tried to remain true to my resolve. I did not receive chemotherapy or radiation, and since tamoxifen was not yet on the scene, I had no further treatment. It was five years before Dr. P. would allow me to have reconstructive surgery. And after a radical mastectomy, this was indeed a painful process. Muscles were taken from my back to replace those that had been cut out of my chest. Recuperation was long and difficult, and I was almost totally immobilized. However, once I looked decent in clothes again and felt like a whole human being, the ordeal was over, and I've never looked back.

Afterword

We have come a long way from the days when "cancer" was a dirty word, and "breast" existed only in the sanctity of the matrimonial bedroom. But I am not sure whether this extreme emancipation in the other direction is as faultless as the former was faulty. With a trend toward sensationalising incidents of malpractice, and so much talk of assertiveness and the need for women to take control of their treatments, is there a place for unsung heroines? Can a woman who bears her predicament in private, who finds peace in trusting her doctors and prefers to be quiescent, survive the intimidation? I raise this issue not as the mother of an oncologist but as a veteran volunteer who, over the years, has seen many different reactions.

I think that what I would like to emphasize is the aspect of privilege. Today women have a choice. If you don't want to talk about it, then don't. There are no rules here. You will not be a lesser person if the inner voice you choose to follow is quieter than the ones resounding about you.

On the other hand, if you do want to discuss your breast cancer and know every last detail about it, nothing should hold you back. Learn. Ask. No question is too stupid or too trivial. Take part in your own treatment, even in your own diagnosis. Insist on a biopsy. Get second, third, or fourth opinions if you want. There is no longer any reason to remain mute and at society's mercy.

Individual human nature is a different story. Fear and ignorance will always seek out opportunity. And even though you are a survivor, or precisely because of it, you represent the natural order of life that no one, of his or her own free will, wants to confront. People will be awkward around you because they don't know what to say. This is not malice but rather their inability to adapt to a paradigm shift. Learning how to reweave the fragile gossamer of personal relationships is, for any survivor, one of breast cancer's more lasting legacies.

Whatever their inclination, many women derive a great deal of strength and comfort from support groups. This is the one community in which everyone is equal. You have neither to explain your emotions nor hide them. It is a place where you can say exactly what's on your mind, without fear of recrimination. For many years now, I have been a volunteer with Hope and Cope and have seen its valuable contribution to the lives of women from all walks of life. A school-bus driver consoles a lawyer. An executive and an artist switch hair-pieces at a meeting, and the entire group is overcome by laughter.

No matter what the situation, we should never lose our ability to have fun. After my own diagnosis, I became determined not to take life, or myself for that matter, too seriously. I wanted a life filled with fun. I wanted to be crazy. It was a relief and a release to allow myself a type of silliness that was both risky and liberating. Now, at this point in my life, I dare to do, and say, as I please.

Just the other day, I was arguing with my bank manager who, even after a forty-year relationship, was sticking to his stubborn, bureaucratic ways and did not want to help me out with a minor detail concerning my husband's business. Each time the answer was no. No, no, no. Sorry. He had to live by the rules. As compensation for his attitude, he sent me a dozen golf balls, knowing that I am an avid golfer. He thought I could be pacified. I picked up the phone and called him right away. "Thank you for the golf balls," I said, "but I want to tell you your balls don't impress me." I even shocked myself. Gert Batist speaking like this? Unthinkable!

The following day, the bank manager called my husband at the office and told him, "Tell your wife, she wins. The papers will be ready tomorrow."

I have one final story to recount. In my English class, we once had a lecture on the great English poet, John Donne. When the professor had finished, he said, "I am done." Everyone booed.

I trust you won't receive me in the same way. For I am done. I wish you happiness, prosperity, and above all, health.

Sister Kathleen Duffin

Montreal, Quebec
Date of birth: August 1, 1939
Date of diagnosis: March 1990

There are not too many aspects of life that I accept unconditionally, without the benefit of careful thought. I suppose you could call this the *yin* and *yang* part of me that prefers to weigh all sides of a situation before forming an opinion. When it comes to taking care of my health, however, there are no ifs, no two points of view. That is why I have been going for regular mammograms ever since I reached "that age" — you know, the one we never truly feel we are at until someone makes a point of reminding us.

In 1989 my annual mammogram was in December, shortly before Christmas. The holidays came and went, and when I heard nothing about my test results, I naturally assumed everything was fine. Three months later I came down with a very bad cold and decided to make an appointment with my family physician. I must tell you that I am not the type who runs to doctors quickly. With three girls in my family growing up, my parents didn't accommodate any type of foolishness, certainly whining. Having been brought up this way, I would have normally let a cold run its course. But this one lingered on.

When I went to see my doctor about it, he diagnosed bronchitis, and, for some reason, also decided to examine my breasts. I don't know why; perhaps he was simply motivated by caution because I had turned fifty recently.

The growth was directly underneath my right nipple, a clandestine weasel that had managed to elude even the spying rays of a mammogram. Fortunately my doctor is a conscientious physician, and his thorough examination detected it. Having made the discovery, he did something that I consider greatly significant. He guided my hand toward the location of the lump — a rather small, hard, round mass — permitting me to feel it and to affirm, so to speak, my connection to it. Instead of treating the lump as an object separate from my body, his action engaged me in the situation right away, establishing the role I would have to play in any medical eventuality. On the surface, his behaviour may appear to have been only a small detail, but as so often happens in life, this seemingly minor gesture was a rich source of inner nourishment.

I got dressed, taking my seat at the opposite end of the doctor's desk, and he quickly settled the issue of the bronchitis with a prescription. The matter of the lump, however, was not as easy. With his elbows planted firmly in front of him, he lowered his head and massaged his temples with his fingertips. He was struggling, formulating in his mind the exact words he wanted to say. Eventually, it was something very simple, short, and matter-of-fact, something to the effect that "we will have to give this a further look." Although he had a very nice way about him, and these words were not intimidating, I immediately thought of breast cancer, every woman's greatest fear. With a sense of urgency, my doctor sent me down the hall to one of his colleagues, who was a surgeon.

A few days later, I found myself in the hospital undergoing a biopsy, the results of which would take about a week to obtain. During this rather extended waiting period, I no doubt felt a certain apprehension, but I did not experience the intense anxiety that often comes with a test of nerves. My intuition told me that it was not my time, and up to that point in my life, my intuition had served me well. When I was young, my sisters attributed this trust in my sixth sense to my so-called "eccentric" side. How many times have I heard them say, "Oh, that's Kay. You know how *she* is!"

Intuition notwithstanding, I breathed a sigh of relief when the surgeon called to say that the tumour was benign. With my health worries behind me, I was able once again to focus all of my energy on my work. I am a college teacher, and spring is always the most stressful time of the year, for teachers as well as students. It is the period before final exams when the school becomes a continuum of nervous commotion.

Barely one week after I had been given a clean bill of health, I was rushing to my office between classes, anticipating the onslaught of students lined up at my door anxiously waiting for answers to their last-minute questions. "Please, Sister Duffin, there's just one thing on page 489 ..." "Do we have to know *even that* material?" "Could you give us just a *small* hint?" "But we skipped over that in class." "Oh, I guess I must have been sick that day."

When I got to my office, the students had not yet arrived. I left the door open to indicate that I was available, and walked over to my desk where a telephone message was waiting for me. It had "URGENT" written across the top in large red letters, underlined. I didn't even have to lower my eyes to see the name of the caller. Instantly I was confronted with a dilemma. If I called the surgeon back and the news was bad, what would I do with my students? They'd be arriving in just a few minutes. On the other hand, if I spent an hour or two with my students, would I be able to reach the surgeon afterwards? As these thoughts flashed through my mind, I couldn't help but imagine the worst and got up from my desk to close the door. Then I dialled the telephone number in front of me.

The surgeon asked that I come over to his office right away. He said that he had some further information — or words to that effect — to discuss with me.

I rushed out of the school — I don't even recall what I told my students — and was sitting in my surgeon's office in under fifteen minutes. Of course he wanted to tell me in person. A review of my case had indicated that the lump was, in fact, malignant.

I stared into space with disbelief, my first reaction being one of dismay. How was this possible? How could they have made such a mistake? At that moment I was more concerned about the misdiagnosis than about the fact that I had breast cancer, and I scared myself with my own speculations about what would have happened had the mistake not been caught. But the surgeon concentrated on the issue at hand, not on the details of the misdiagnosis. He said that because the lump was relatively small and unlikely to have metastasized, I could probably get away with a partial mastectomy followed by radiation treatments.

Seven years ago, the word "lumpectomy" did not exist. Everything was a mastectomy; differences were only a matter of degree: radical, modified, total, partial. As a teacher I have always emphasized that imagery and suggestion are the essence of language. While it is quite true that a rose is a rose by any other name, a "prickle-stemmed enfoldment" will not inspire our senses in the same way. By the same token, lumpectomy is a softer and more subtle word than mastectomy, evoking the prospect of a less dramatic illness. So this subtlety, however it has come about, is definitely an improvement from the days when I was diagnosed.

Nonetheless, I felt as if I were in a foreign world, listening to my doctor compose the oddest sentences. The individual words were familiar: Estrogen ... receptor ... positive ... and radiation ... as adjuvant ... therapy ... and so on. But I had never heard them side by side before.

Then the surgeon told me to think everything over. First, there was the timing to consider, although I didn't have much latitude in that regard. A few weeks perhaps. And then there was the issue of the surgery itself — whether or not I would submit to a total mastectomy.

All the while, my mind was jumping from one thought to the next, scrambling to anchor itself somewhere. Suddenly, there were so many issues to deal with. And my students! With still a few weeks left in the semester, I would need to find teachers to cover my religious-studies and humanities classes.

Before reaching any decision, I made up my mind to go to a larger hospital for a second opinion, on the off chance that bigger might be better. The second surgeon explained in detail the procedures that were followed at his hospital. My case would be brought up — along with every other newly diagnosed case that week — and presented to a team of doctors who would then decide on the type of surgery and course of treatment that was right for me. The process sounded very complex, and I felt uncomfortable with it, so even as the second surgeon was speaking, I made up my mind to go with the first one. His disposition was both peaceful and reassuring, despite the misdiagnosis. That was not his fault. I knew that. Furthermore, I was very familiar with his hospital and liked it. It is one of the smaller ones in Montreal with a strong sense of community, and many Sisters go there.

Having made my first major decision, I was so proud of myself that I decided I deserved a reward. I went for a leisurely stroll on the prettiest commercial street in the neighbourhood, my version of a shopping spree. I was walking along Queen Mary Road when I spotted a bookstore. Inside, in a completely unrelated section, I saw a book at eye level, almost as if I were meant to find it. It was called *Surviving Breast Cancer*, by Carol Spearin McCauley, and I began reading it immediately. Like a detective novel, it engaged my curiosity from the start, except that the suspense revolved around me and my particular case, and the outcome of my own story was what had to be resolved. I couldn't put it down.

On my way back home, I walked slowly, deeply immersed in a new world of information, barely lifting my head from the pages. The only thing that interrupted my concentration was the honking of approaching cars, but I paid no attention. I'm a driver myself, so I know that Montrealers honk too much. Or maybe I really was in harm's way. I don't recall.

The book was my gateway into the mysterious expanse that is the universe of cancer. I easily identified my own circumstances and focused on the prognosis. The tumour had been caught at an early stage, and the cure rate was above ninety percent. Later that evening, as I turned over the last page, I felt that I had a lot going for me. I became peaceful about my situation, and in time this quiescence would come to permeate my entire cancer experience. Certainly there were times along the way when I was frightened, but never so frightened as to think that I would not recover.

In fact, during my five-month sojourn towards recovery, I recall having had only one big bout of anger. That happened on the day I had to go back to see my surgeon — the day I was told about the misdiagnosis. My middle sister, Lois, and I had planned to go to Ireland in the summer, and we'd had a date for that very same day to price out some possibilities. But instead of the travel agent, I saw a breast surgeon; instead of holiday options, I was given treatment alternatives; and instead of being in Ireland for three weeks, I would be in radiation for six. These things made me angry.

Overall, however, the emotions that accompany grave circumstances could not taunt me into pessimistic digressions. From the outset, I had always had a sense that there was a deliberate reason for my bronchitis. I could have taken care of a common cold on my own with a few aspirins and chicken soup. But bronchitis led me to the doctor who examined my breasts. The fact that the malignancy had been detected at such an early stage had not, I concluded, been a random event.

But I continued to be bothered by the misdiagnosis and had to get the whole story to satisfy myself. My search led me straight down to the records office of the hospital. I told them that I wanted to know who had read my X-rays and who had found the cancer. Because it was a rather small hospital, the information was easy to obtain. Then, X-rays in hand, I went to see the radiologist. She was an American, in Montreal only temporarily on a brief exchange. She informed me that all biopsy cases are reviewed by a "tumour board," just as it had been explained to me at the larger hospital where I had gone for a second opinion. Ironically, the very procedure that had seemed to me too complex and unreliable had saved me from a potential crisis. The results, I learned, are read to the board in the manner of a roll-call: Smith — benign; Jones — malignant; Cooper — benign; Duffin — benign. And on Duffin, she had interjected, "Oh, just a minute."

She had seen a shadow on my X-ray that the others had overlooked because it had a number of characteristics not normally associated with a malignancy. Fortunately, it was a shadow that she had come across a few times before. Since pathology still had my tissue culture, the hospital was able to perform further tests, eventually producing the positive diagnosis.

After hearing this, I didn't know how to appropriately thank the person whose intervention may have saved my life. I cannot remember exactly what I said, but I will certainly never forget her response. While very gracious, she maintained that she had just been "doing her job."

After all was said and done, I knew how the mistake had been discovered, but I still wasn't sure how it had been made. I had a nagging thought that wouldn't go away — what if this particular radiologist hadn't been there that day? Or perhaps I just needed closure and expected it in the form of an apology.

More than once, a student has come to me after receiving a graded exam to show me that I've marked an answer wrong when in fact it was right. In every instance I have corrected the grade, thanked the student for bringing it to my attention, and expressed my remorse. I think this is a big issue for a lot of people — admitting having made a mistake. When it came to the error made in my case, perhaps I was expecting the same type of behaviour that I require of myself. I simply needed someone to say to me, "we are sorry." But this never happened. Now, having weighed the issue in my mind many times, I've concluded that it really doesn't matter. The important thing is that my cancer was caught at an early stage and that the tumour was small.

The surgeon said that if all went well, he would make the incision in the same spot that he had performed the biopsy, in order to avoid creating two separate scars on my breast. He also promised to leave my nipple intact, although it would shift positions slightly. I was comforted by this type of thoughtfulness and considered myself lucky, because I know there can be misconceptions about the importance of physical integrity to religious men and women.

My own encounters with compassion, however, were not restricted to this isolated event. And except for one quarrelsome incident at an appointment with the oncologist, I met with sensitivity in the medical community, over and over again.

Consider this act of kindness, for example. I entered the hospital the week before Easter — Passion week. When I went to see the admissions clerk, she looked at my insurance contract and told me that I was only entitled to double occupancy. With this understanding, she filled out the necessary forms and gave them to me to sign. I did, and handed them back to her. As she reviewed the papers, she must have recognized the "cnd" — standing for Congregation Notre Dame — that I write as part of my signature, and suddenly looked up at me. "Seeing as this is holy week," she said, "you might want to have a room all to yourself, Sister Duffin. It is not very large, and it's at the end of the corridor, but if you want to have it, you're most welcome." Well, that room was just fine. True, it was no larger than a closet, but all I needed was a bed and a bathroom, and since I am not a television watcher, I lacked nothing.

On the morning of my operation, the surgeon wanted my permission to do whatever was necessary once I was on the operating table. Of course I knew what that meant. And because I had confidence in him I agreed. Just as there are times when you must insist on your participation in the medical process, questioning and probing your doctor's decisions, I think there are also times when you must trust that the doctor knows what he or she is doing. My surgery was this moment of trust, and that trust was not unjustified.

On April 9, 1990, the tumour was removed by means of a partial mastectomy, and a few days later, I found out that my lymph nodes were clear.

At my first appointment with the oncologist, I was expecting to discuss the details of my combined radiation/tamoxifen treatment, which the surgeon had explained to me only in very broad terms. Less than thirty seconds into the visit, the oncologist said, "We're not so sure that you *will* get tamoxifen." I was astonished. He then proceeded to tell me that my name would go into a central pool, in the United States no less, and that on a basis of random selection I would either receive tamoxifen or not. We would only find out a few years down the road if the consequences were to my benefit. I later learned that this is called a protocol.

Puzzled by this turn of events, I replied, really quite naïvely, "But my surgeon told me I would be taking tamoxifen." How interesting. There I was, asking for it, feeling like a child disappointed by a broken promise.

The oncologist became openly agitated and used a most provocative tone, saying, "I didn't tell your surgeon where to cut, did I?" He was clearly implying that, by the same token, the surgeon had no right to interfere in his oncological matters. Now in view of the fact that it was *my* life at stake, I got annoyed and retorted brusquely, "This is *my* cancer and *my* body, and I will be the one to decide." It came out just like that! I couldn't believe what I was saying. All of my adult life I have spoken with reservation and courtesy. But on this occasion it seemed that my mouth had decided to take off on its own. I am tempted to attribute this to the Irish in me, and my friends would probably agree. When pushed hard enough I, too, can lose my temper.

As women, the majority of us have been brought up to respect all forms of authority, particularly if it's patriarchal. Many of us find confrontations with physicians — especially male doctors — uncomfortable, and we avoid them. But we have to learn to stand up for ourselves.

This encounter with the oncologist is precisely the type of situation where a woman shouldn't take a doctor's word for granted, where she should take responsibility for herself. Whether it's your intuition, your body, your newly acquired knowledge of cancer, or your Irish blood talking, listen to it. And if you don't want to take part in a protocol, all you have to do is say no. It may be necessary to repeat yourself once or twice, but sooner or later you will be heard. In the end, I received the tamoxifen, just as I had requested.

***

Perhaps you are wondering to what extent my vocation helped me get through the rough spots. The answer is that I have accumulated many invaluable tools over the past thirty-five years, and that I relied on my faith no more and no less in this situation than I have in any other. Faith is a non-discriminatory part of my existence, and I live with God each and every moment. Meditation has been part of my daily life since 1960 when I joined the Community. And I have always been a reflective individual. So, as I contemplated this business of living and dying, my years of trying to be open to God's will in my life paid off. Fear — the type of fear that blots out all hope — never stood a chance. Often, however, I did bring the issue to prayer.

Then, too, I was lucky in the amount of emotional support available to me. At the time of my diagnosis, I was living on the Villa Maria grounds in a pleasant French community, of which several Sisters were long-term breast cancer survivors. The fact that they were there, among the living, was heartening evidence that I could fight this disease and win. And since these Sisters are also my friends, they were always there for me, especially when I felt the most vulnerable.

I will not be so presumptuous as to deny the possibility that I was not fully in touch with what was going on, or indeed, that I didn't want to be in touch. My friend Jane, who is a psychologist, told me on more than one occasion that I wasn't dealing with my illness. She expected me to be upset, and I simply replied that she couldn't force me. One summer afternoon, after I had returned from radiation, she was sitting with me in the grass on the Villa grounds when she burst out impatiently, "Would you stop smiling Kay, you have cancer!"

"I can't help it," I told her. "You know me. I'm a smiler, not a frowner." I suppose this sums up my attitude.

But it would be a misconception for you to think that my being a Sister means that I have it "all figured out." For as long as I can remember, changes have been taking place all around me, in all three spheres of my life — vocational, professional and personal. And change can often create deep internal conflicts, the resolutions of which are neither clear nor imminent.

When I joined the Community, we were halfway through the pontificate of John XXIII. It was a time of extreme flux, with the Vatican embarking on a process intended to open up theology. Centuries-old traditions were being re-evaluated. Formulas and discipline, which had existed for hundreds of years, were being revised. All religious men and women had to come to terms with the enormity of these changes.

Over the years, confusion and disillusion about the reforms in the Community have been so pervasive that many women who entered with me have decided to leave. Yet I have stayed my course, struggling to work things through, and my life has been full indeed. This doesn't mean that I did not question things. I certainly did. But my main consideration was not whether the Church could handle my questioning. It was God I was concerned about.

Today, certain ethical issues impact the Church at its core, and these are very big questions for me. And because I am an educator, I have to deal with them on two levels. First, I have my own personal views to consider, and second, I must allow the opinions of others — my students — to enter the debate. The convergence of these two facets of my life lends my existence a colourful but complex fabric.

What does any of this have to do with my cancer experience? Let me answer in this way.

My life has been full of challenges, which means that as a woman and a member of a religious community I have had to learn how to adapt and live through them. From this point of view, breast cancer was my peak experience. When I examined how cancer fit into the mystery of my life's journey, I saw it as an opportunity to carry me into a richer dimension of reflection and self-examination.

Breast cancer caused me to see things according to a different pattern. I look more deeply and more honestly at issues now. I am aware that everything evolves, that everything takes time. I realize that my desire to have things happen more quickly isn't going to make them happen more quickly. And this doesn't get to me as much any more. My attitude is different. It is not that I don't feel as passionately about things as I did when I was younger, it is simply that my reaction to them has changed. I have become somewhat more patient, maybe a little calmer, less strident about some of the issues that are relevant in my life. I have learned to discern. That is a spiritual term we use a lot — the discernment of spirits. And since I have always had a tendency to work myself hard, I have also had to learn to say "no."

***

I was diagnosed with breast cancer at the age of fifty. At the time, I never thought of myself as middle-aged, let alone troubled by the issue of my mortality. I had not become the person who, as a child, I had always imagined older people to be. I have particular memories of Thursday nights, the only time of the week we were allowed to listen to the radio. My favourite show was called *House on the Hill*. It was sponsored by Ponds facial cream and the commercial used to say, "At twenty-five a woman begins to lose the natural oil of her skin." Twenty-five, I thought to myself. That's so old! And when my mother died at forty-eight, I remember people at the wake commenting, "She was so young." But to me, forty-eight was old.

Not surprisingly, when *I* reached twenty-five, and forty-eight, and fifty, I was still young. I thought young. And I always believed I would live until eighty or eight-five. After breast cancer, I paused. Perhaps I had been wrong. To a certain extent, we all take the routine of life for granted, and this particular illness makes one take stock. You become privy to a heightened awareness of your own existence, of the truth that you are part of a whole that is larger than yourself and your environs. In essence, you become privileged by this awareness. I sensed the rarity of this privilege and the opportunity it gave me to rediscover my individuality, my purpose, and my relationship with God.

As a postscript to this story, I would like to add that during the course of our relationship, which has lasted now close to eight years, the oncologist and I have become good friends. Whenever I see him, whether every three months, as I did in the beginning, or on a six-month basis, as I do today, he always turns the visit into a discussion about my mental well-being. He enquires about my current course-load at work, my holiday plans — whether or not I am taking summer vacation or time off during the Christmas period — and the extent of my commitments to the Community, as well as to my personal life. It has occurred to me that, being of Spanish origin, he is probably very knowledgable about the intense work habits of religious men and women. He knows me well enough to realize that I, too, have a tendency to over-extend myself, and he has taken it upon himself to be my guardian, of sorts.

Afterword

I grew up in a faith-filled, Irish-Catholic family, the eldest of three girls. Our mother died when I was eighteen, which meant that I had to learn early on, and quite suddenly, to be independent and make my own decisions. These things have stayed with me throughout my life.

I made my most significant decision at the age of twenty-one when I chose to enter the Community, fully aware of the challenges involved. I knew the other side, and what I would be giving up, and realized the consequences should my decision turn out to be the wrong one.

I chose to enter the Congregation of Notre Dame because it was a teaching Order (founded by Marguerite Bourgeois in 1660). As much as it appealed to my strong sense of faith, it also fulfilled my desire to perform work of value to society at large. Later, I obtained an undergraduate degree in English literature and began my teaching career. That was over thirty years ago.

My life's journey has not led me away from my original commitment; instead it has led me, I hope, in the direction of enhanced wisdom. I have a sense that things are happening in my life that would have been wasted on me had they occurred earlier.

Having to embrace the fact of my own mortality made me appreciate my gifts — that each day itself is a gift. Even after eight years, it still challenges me to be my *best* self, to focus on the quality of life rather than the inevitability of death.

The ability to insulate ourselves against the emotional turmoil of a breast cancer diagnosis is really not the issue in my view. What *is* important is for each of us to allow our own version of these feelings to unfold, working our way through each stage and letting it run its course. Eventually the pain will pass, for the capacity of the human spirit to heal itself is limitless.

This may be an awful thing to say, but the summer of 1990 turned out to be a truly wonderful one. I was surrounded by friendship and care, I had lunch served to me every day after my radiation treatments at the hospital, and even though I was tired, I was able to relax and read, watch the children play, listen to the birds and bask in the glow of idyllic, sunny afternoons. I felt like a little girl again, carefree, playing in the grass.

Perhaps my personal evolution can be attributed, in part, to the passage of time, to the fact that I am entering a more serene, mature phase in my life. But I would like to believe that breast cancer has been a means, as have all the experiences in my life, of growing, like Jesus, in wisdom and age and grace.

Sophie LeBlanc

Montreal, Quebec
Date of birth: August 3, 1966
Date of diagnosis: October 12, 1994

"True prayer and love are really learned in the hour when prayer becomes impossible and your heart turns to stone." These words were written by Thomas Merton, the twentieth-century monk and philosopher who, towards the end of his life, was referred to as *geshe* — learned lama — by the Dalai Lama of Tibet. I chose this passage from Merton's opus, *Seeds of Contemplation*, because it is particularly apt for those of us who have suffered the pain of a breast cancer diagnosis and who, as survivors, continue to live with it, forever joined to one another in spirit.

***

I first felt a lump in my breast in July 1993. As it wasn't very large I wasn't too concerned, and postponed having it looked at until September, during my annual check-up with my family physician. After examining me, the doctor said that the lump looked like a cyst, but being a cautious person, she decided to have me see a breast specialist. She made the appointment while I was still in her office. It would be in two months.

By the time I saw the specialist in December, the lump had grown, probably to about three centimetres. The doctor looked at it, felt it, and examined me, but performed no diagnostic tests. He reassured me that it was only a fibro adenoma and told me to come back in three months. In fact, he was so sure of his diagnosis that he didn't even do a needle biopsy or send me for a mammogram. "BIG Mistake," as Julia Roberts says in *Pretty*

Woman. Yes, doctors make mistakes too, but in the world of medicine these can be very costly.

I followed the surgeon's instructions and exactly three months later called for another appointment. As before, I was told that I would have to wait. I didn't end up returning to the surgeon until May, five months after he had first seen me, and almost one year since I'd first noticed the lump.

Even though I was aware that the lump was growing, I didn't react to this delay with panic. I had many reasons for choosing to respond casually to my condition. My family doctor was reliable and had always referred me to excellent specialists, which meant that I had faith in the surgeon's initial judgement. More importantly, there were a lot of things happening in my life. I was doing a combined Masters and Ph.D degree in education, I was a freelance researcher for television, I had a lot of family issues to deal with — problems in my personal relationships — and I had a little girl who commandeered all of my remaining attention. I was drained on all fronts — physically, emotionally, and intellectually. And let's face it, when you're twenty-seven years old, you don't feel like hearing you have cancer. So when they insist that you don't, you tend to believe them.

In May, during that second appointment with the specialist, however, I did attempt to convince him that a biopsy made sense. Once again, I was reassured that the procedure was unnecessary. I was young, there was no history of breast cancer in my family, I had given birth at an early age and, all told, I had none of the established risk-factors associated with this disease. The surgeon saw no need for a biopsy. But by now a little voice inside my head had emerged: what about the fact that the lump is growing? Still, I tried to be deaf to it.

September of 1994 marked my next annual check-up with my family physician. After we had dispensed with the routine pap smear and a general conversation about diet and lifestyle, I almost forgot to show her my breast. Fourteen months had passed since the lump first appeared, and I could see the shock on her face as she looked at it; the lump was so large that my breast had changed shape. She immediately called the specialist and arranged for me to see him the following morning.

This was my third visit to the breast surgeon, and I noticed right away that his tone was different. What stands out most in my mind is his particular choice of words. After he, too, had been visibly shaken by what he saw, he

said quite emphatically, "We are going to give it all the respect it deserves."
What a strange choice of words, I thought. "It," rather than "me." I shouldn't
have been surprised. A surgeon's primary relationship is with body tissue, not
the soul.

From that point on, everything happened very quickly. I had three tests in
a row — a mammogram, an ultrasound, and a thermogram. And because of
the reaction I was getting from the technicians and physicians around me, I had
a disturbing premonition. They may as well have been waving placards in my
face. Their body language said it all. I had cancer.

***

Two years earlier, I had lost my best friend in a car accident, and this terrible
tragedy had marked the beginning of a downward slide. On every front, my life
seemed to go from bad to worse. At the end I was so trapped by circumstances
that I felt I had lost control over everything that was happening to me.

Over the years I had become very adept at "busying" — keeping busy
doing this, doing that. My daily life had become dedicated to defining my
identity through busyness, in order to keep up with my own self-image. It had
become necessary for me to take on many roles, and no one would deny that I
had fashioned myself into something of a superwoman. I was wife, mother,
career professional, confidant to friends, graduate student, hostess, and an
assortment of additional personas required of me by a variety of situations.
Naturally, in each of these roles I had to give away a part of myself, so I was
defined not only by the roles I played, but by how much I was able to give.
Within this life there was no room for Sophie, whomever she was.

I had to live up to the standards expected of me, the most important of which
were my own. And I had taught my community to expect of me the same level
of commitment that I expected of myself. Since the concept of failure was not
part of my mind-set, I found myself trying harder and harder, giving more and
more, in order to satisfy my perfectionist bent. As a freelancer I always had to
hustle, so I was either looking for a contract or working on one. In addition, I
was finishing my Master's thesis, chauffering my daughter, preparing to host
dinner parties in the evening, living it up until past midnight, getting four hours
of restless sleep, and starting all over again the next day.

My energy levels had always been very high, and I pushed myself beyond
my physical capabilities. I would forge ahead when I felt completely drained,

unmindful of any warning signs my body might be trying to give me. I was invincible, you see. Everybody told me so.

Eventually, the intensity of my lifestyle caught up with me, and many times I hit bottom while outwardly giving the impression that I was on top of things. Then, when I could no longer keep up pretenses and was sinking further and further into the darkness, people around me reacted the way I had trained them to. Sophie's okay, they said. Sophie will make it. Sophie never falls apart. Sophie is a go-getter. Sophie will bounce back in no time.

I can't really say that no one offered to help. Almost everyone did, but I was unable to receive their help because I didn't know how. I knew only how to give. That was who I was — the giver. I think this is called "misguided self-sacrifice" or "martyr syndrome" or some such thing.

I had to escape and I saw only one way out. In all likelihood, a less desperate woman would have merely wished to get sick. But in this regard, too, I had high standards. It was all or nothing. So I wished myself dead. I wished and wished and wished.

Now, that wish was within my grasp. In a matter of one week, I had gone from perfect health to the prospect of losing a body part. But what freaked me out the most was the thought of being anaesthetized for the operation. It was the procedure itself that scared me, not the cancer. I was not yet ready to be scared of that.

On October 19, 1994, at ten o'clock in the morning, they wheeled me into the amphitheatre for a partial mastectomy. I didn't know it at the time, but my surgeon had just received the results of my bone scan. The cancer had metastasized.

When I spoke with him afterward, I must admit that he seemed to feel very badly about the situation. He was fully conscious of the fact that he had made a mistake, and he half-heartedly acknowledged it. But this was a poor consolation prize. I was terminal, and he had signed my death sentence. (He hadn't even bothered to do a good job, and my scar is about one inch thick and six inches wide, spanning almost half my chest.)

In my mind, the worst part was not that he had missed the initial diagnosis, but that when I had asked him specific questions about it, he had lied to me. And from my point of view, his real mistake was that he had trusted his own judgement too much. He had been so arrogant that he never gave a thought to confirming his diagnosis, either the first time I went to see him or the second, when he clearly could see that the lump had grown. There is a dangerously fine line between the self-confidence necessary to trust your own judgement and an arrogance that impels you to preclude any opinion but your own.

During our post-op conversation, he gave me only scant bits of information, revealing in part that I would now have to be examined by an oncology committee. Little did I know what this would entail.

I met the committee four days before Hallowe'en — rather fitting when I consider what was to come. I was handed one of those blue hospital gowns — I've always detested those things — and placed on a bed in a very tiny room. The door was shut. Of course I knew that on the other side they were all huddled together, discussing my case. There were five or six oncologists and countless radiologists, surgeons, nurses, residents, and medical students. All of a sudden the door opened, and I had a throng of people staring at me. There must have been at least twenty-five of them. The scene resembled a burlesque. With everyone hovering over me, I felt like the body in Rembrandt's "Anatomy Lesson of Dr. Tulp." In response to this absurdity, I put on the biggest smile I could muster and said in a hearty voice, "Well HELLO everybody! Welcome ..." They all started laughing and unfortunately didn't hear the rest, "... to my nightmare."

The atmosphere in the room was tense. I was a case, a curiosity, the bearded woman, a twenty-eight-year-old with no genetic condition and Stage IV metastatic breast cancer. Perhaps it was due to my status as a case-study, because I made them somewhat uncomfortable, that I thought it was incumbent upon me to break the ice. Or maybe I simply used humour as a means of masking the truth. I have always been good at that.

A short little fellow began asking me hundreds of seemingly irrelevant questions: Had I suffered a lot of bike accidents as a child? Did I remember falling down a lot? Had I been hit by anyone? He must have been attempting to account for the lesions in my bones. I was surprised by his intense curiousity, and it caught me off guard. But later I realized that I prefer my doctors serious, even panicky, because this makes them act quickly. Seriousness means complete dedication to my cause. If it happens that a panic is for nothing, well then nothing is lost. I've learned my lesson with doctors who assume too much, who do not take complaints in earnest, and I never want to repeat the experience I had with my surgeon. One close encounter of that kind was enough.

Another character approaching through the crowd began tugging at the sleeves of my gown, trying to take a peek at my breast. He never said a word, just pulled a little and peeked a little, hoping I wouldn't notice. Finally I got fed up. "Who are you?" I asked, exasperated. He introduced himself as Doctor So-and-So and looked at me rather squeamishly. "Can I examine you?" he said. "Well yeah," I replied, "all you have to do is ask. I don't bite."

In the final analysis, it comes down to this. I know it was necessary to examine me. I know they had to evaluate my physical condition in order to determine my treatment alternatives. But there must be a better way to achieve the same end. So here's a challenge to the medical community. Develop a more sensitive, more humane process for assessing late-stage breast cancer patients, because the current procedure is nothing short of barbaric.

***

After the committee was through with me, the surgeon said that the chief oncologist would be the one to give me the official diagnosis. Not many women liked this man, he warned, because he was extremely staid and often appeared to be dispassionate. I told him that I would form my own opinion, thank you.

The moment I saw the oncologist, I remembered him from my meeting with the committee. He was very reserved and almost shy, with an air of sincere compassion about him. He confirmed that I had Stage IV breast cancer, metastasized to the bones, and told me it was incurable. I had two choices for treatment. The first was regular chemotherapy. And because I was young and had never had chemo before, the chances of remission were good. That would give me two years. Then, after a recurrence, I would get chemo again, which would add another year and a half, bringing my total future to roughly four years. It was most bizarre to see elementary-school arithmetic applied in this way, since I had never thought of death and math in the same context before.

He then went on to explain my second option. This entailed a protocol — high dose chemotherapy with two bone-marrow transplants. It was still in the experimental stage and only available in Montreal at one hospital. Moreover, because of the side effects, this treatment would require extended hospitalization with a minimum stay of 130 days. The greatest shock, however, was being told that the treatments would make me sterile. Until then I hadn't been sure whether I wanted to have more kids or not, but now it seemed the decision might be made for me, and I wasn't prepared for it. Somehow the finality suggested by this second option was more distressing than the diagnosis itself.

The more I asked, the more information the oncologist offered. I was grateful for his honesty and told him I needed some time to think about it. He understood. I had to be very sure and very comfortable with my decision. And he made it clear that it *would be* my decision.

I ended the session by telling him what I had heard of his terrible reputation. No wonder. He always had to play the bad guy, the bearer of bad news. "So I will call you Dr. Badnews from now on," I said, pleased with another successful attempt at humour, or so I thought. It was a while before I realized that the doctor was not living very well with this tag, and that he hadn't said otherwise out of kindness to me. But one day, when I introduced him to a friend as "Dr. Badnews," I saw the hurt in his eyes and knew that my joke had run its course.

Although I was leaning toward the protocol, I wasn't sure I could handle the additional element of anxiety it would entail. It would be necessary to change hospitals, go to a different oncologist, and face a new team of doctors. I would have barely completed my rite of passage from lab mouse to human being when the cage doors would be swung wide open once again, ushering me back inside.

I decided to meet with the protocol team's psychiatrist, hoping to regain some of the faith I had lost in medicine. After all, could one blame me? Just look at my history, I said — the surgeon's arrogance, the misdiagnosis, its consequences, the final diagnosis, the oncology committee, my status as a medical case, and my pending infertility. Considering what lay ahead, I had to believe that taking part in the protocol was the best thing for me and that the doctors really knew what they were doing. I had to renew my confidence in the system because without it I could not conceive of undergoing any type of treatment at all. My intuition was telling me that this would be the right thing to do, but I had to be sure. These were complex issues to resolve. In fact, when it comes to cancer, we all have to learn, very quickly, that there are no simple issues, no clear-cut answers.

Next, I went to see the oncologist in charge of the protocol, and I must admit that I entered his office a very angry woman. By then, given the gravity of my situation and the harrowing treatment I had endured, my ruling emotion was rage. I lived with it, slept with it, and awoke with it. For a long time after my surgery, I had visualized the tumour as my rage and had tried to convince myself that with its removal, the rage had also been cut out of my body. But it hadn't. I was aggressive, and Dr. S. responded in kind. He was abrupt. He threw statistics at me. And facts. And probabilities. But I wanted reassurances. "I am not a statistic," I said over and over again. Then he would repeat the facts, and I would repeat my stance. I was not one of one hundred; I was one of one.

I left the room in worse condition than when I entered it. Yes, the anger was still there, but now I was also beaten and broken. If I decided to join the protocol, how was I going to deal with this man for a year? We would be battling one another the whole time.

I think I desperately wanted him to acknowledge the psychological impact of the various procedures, because it was on that level that I would need him to relate to me. This was the man who would hold my life in his hands, who would make every single decision about my body, what chemicals would enter it and how to treat the effects. This was the man in charge of food, drink, visitors, whom I could see, whom I could touch. This was the man in charge of everything.

After that first meeting with Dr. S., I decided to seek out second and third opinions. As I sat in front of each successive doctor and handed over my charts, they gave me the same look, the one I had seen many times but had not yet acquired the courage to acknowledge. The look that said, "Oh my God, she's dead."

Both doctors were forthright and said the same thing: two to five years. My treatment options were exactly what I had been told.

Of all the doctors I had met up to that point, it was the second of these oncologists who influenced me the most. He was very human, very generous with his emotions, and understood that I had lost my balance. "So you don't give me much of a chance either," I stated, ruefully. He asked what made me think that, and I replied that I had become very good at reading faces. Well,

I was wrong in trying to put words in his mouth, for he responded with a long monologue. It went something like this:

"You know, Sophie, you're a bit too young to be my wife, a bit too old to be my daughter, and I don't have any mistresses. But probably all the doctors you went to see are men. You could be *their* wives, *their* daughters, and *their* mistresses. Without exception, we all relate to that. Take my word for it. This is why we try our best in every situation, with every woman. We just have different ways of showing it. As for statistics, you are the only statistic that exists. We cannot swear that you are *not* going to make it, and we cannot swear that you *are* going to make it. And if you do decide to choose something experimental, just make sure it is recorded. Make sure it will be a published protocol and that you will be data, so that medicine will not lose what you will do. If it works, we'll know. If it doesn't work, we'll know. In either case, you will have contributed to science and made a difference in the world."

I hadn't thought of it this way before, and his words infiltrated a niche in my psyche. This was the legacy I wanted to leave.

When I informed the protocol oncologist of my decision to participate in his experimental procedures, he appeared to be genuinely happy — I like to think not only on his own behalf but on mine as well. And his attitude toward me changed almost immediately. The abrasive detachment was gone. In its place, I found a caring human being, a physician committed to his patients with intensity and devotion. He moved mountains for me when he had to. No stone was left unturned. When he worried, I worried. When he didn't worry, neither did I. And, once I had become used to his sense of humour, I was able to have lots of fun with him.

During the entire span of our association, we have never spoken about our first, rather unpleasant, encounter. I realize now that he simply wanted to give me a slap in the face, as if to say, "Hey, this is not a cold you're running here. You have cancer. It is serious, and we have to do something about it. Here is what I can do."

Our relationship has matured into one of mutual respect, understanding and kindness, just as I had wanted. We have become very close. But before I give you the wrong impression, let me say that this has not been a fairy tale. Dr. S. was always very honest, even about his limited success rate, before I signed up. I therefore had to deal with the fact that I might not make it, despite the painful and aggressive procedures that lay ahead of me.

Unfortunately, because experimental protocols must first be approved, I was unable to begin treatment right away. Meanwhile, my bones were deteriorating, even though I wasn't experiencing a lot of pain. Then, when my neck began to hurt, everyone suddenly became extremely worried. It turned out to be a collapsed vertebrae, and I had to wear a surgical collar for two months. This was all a bit too much for Dr. S., and he immediately went into action. He literally stopped everything, turned everybody upside down for me, and cut through the bureaucratic tape with the sharp edge of his will. He received approval for me to begin the protocol ahead of schedule, on compassionate grounds.

My treatments began on March 31, 1995. The protocol entailed six cycles of intensive chemotherapy, one cycle per month, to prepare my body for the two bone-marrow transplants. The transplants were then followed by radiation for six weeks. I would spend the remainder of 1995 in the hospital, either as an in-patient for two to three weeks at a time, or as an out-patient, occasionally winding up back in emergency for one reason or another.

You are probably wondering why, if I had wanted to die, I signed up for the protocol in the first place, or decided to undergo any type of treatment at all.

As I reflect on it today, I think I know the answer. Wishing for death provided the safest means of escape because being dead and wishing it are not, after all, the same thing. In a sense, the wish allowed me to have it both ways. The wish became the actual escape, allowing me to exist in a state of virtual death.

When the breast cancer diagnosis came along, it instantly removed the element of safety from my clever escape device. The ensuing confrontation between what was virtual and what was actual must have aroused my instinct for survival.

Wishing for death was also the most dishonest way of getting rid of my problems, since it eliminated any need to examine myself and find another way out, a less drastic option. The diagnosis exposed this dishonesty, and I was forced to choose between either facing myself and finding an alternate route or remaining in the comfort of self-deceit and dying. At first I didn't want to choose and went around saying that I didn't care if I lived or died.

Then, without warning, I felt conflicting emotions vying for my attention. From the visceral depths of a panic attack, I would switch to the opposite extreme. Although aware that I had a grave medical condition, I began taking the news very lightly. No one around me could understand why I was constantly laughing and making jokes, seemingly carefree. I think I must have also gone into denial, hiding in the comfort of lightheartedness. Once denial was no longer an issue, I quickly entered the"why me" phase, and got out of it just as fast. I had a hundred explanations for what had happened to me, and they were all to my intellectual satisfaction. Put simply, I had set myself up. For a time,"if only" was my favourite thought, and I became convinced that I alone had brought the cancer upon myself.

Immediately after choosing to participate in the protocol, I again met with the team psychiatrist, and told him that I had three problems. First, I was scared more of the treatments than of the disease. Second, it was not so bad to have cancer because I would finally be able to take a break. And third, I didn't know how I would endure being in hospital for a period of one year. Dr. V. looked at me quite sombrely and said, "You're right, Sophie, you do have problems. But I think there are more than three."

As it turned out, I had a lot of work ahead of me, and in the beginning I spent a great deal of energy on "taming." I had to tame my mind, my environment, my relationships, and every aspect of my life that previously had been devoted to anger.

Dr. V. also prodded me with frequent wake-up calls. He always had good one-liners with which to shake me up, such as, "Sophie, you have a wall in front of you. You're running straight into it, and you are going to die." He'd come up with sobering questions, frighteningly blunt: "Will you have to die, Sophie LeBlanc, to show that you exist?" In the black and white of the paper on which you are reading this, Dr. V. might seem very harsh, perhaps even cruel, but his words were my cod-liver oil. I had to swallow them before I could get better.

Unfortunately, there are no guidelines, no rules, no twelve-step methods for dealing with a terminal diagnosis. So I hung on to Dr. V. as if my life depended on him. And in many ways it did. I gradually regained my reverence for life and, assisted by other events that occurred at that time, soon found myself embarking on a quest for self-discovery.

There was almost a half-year gap between my partial mastectomy and the date I entered the hospital to begin the protocol. And since I now understand that nothing happens without a reason, the point of this delay is quite clear. I had two diseases to cure. The hospital was responsible for healing my body. But I had sole ownership of the process by which I would heal my spirit. This five-month window gave me the opportunity to do just that. I never would have been able to withstand the physical effects of the protocol with a shattered spirit.

My internal restoration followed an erratic but persistent course, and the insights I gained along the way eventually widened into a beautiful, winding path, leading to *tathagatagarbha* — the essence of Buddhism.

***

As a teenager I had been fascinated by Tibet, and between the ages of fourteen and eighteen, I sought out every piece of information I could find, from any possible source. I read what was available at the library, I went to documentary movies and photography exhibits, but still I wasn't sated. At that time I also began looking into Buddhism, but I was a Christian then and my traditional upbringing triumphed. Later, at university, I delved into philosophy, which further aroused my interest in the essence of the human soul.

Although cut short, these early excursions into foreign consciousness were not lost to me. I had become sidetracked by life, but the imprints remained. The memories of my Tibetan experience began to resurface at the same time that Dr. V. was helping me restore my will to live.

The winter of 1994 was packed with providence. The first cancer patient I talked to was the friend of a friend, a survivor who had beaten the odds. Diagnosed with lung cancer in 1990, she had been given ten months to live. As she described her entire life experience to me, her words revealed a path very similar to my own. Before her diagnosis, she too had been at the end of her rope and had wanted to die. Furthermore, she hadn't believed in remission because she had lost a sister to cancer. News of her illness forced her to confront herself. If I want to die, she thought, here is the road right in front of me. It's all mine. I won't take any treatments. I'll just get on that road, in and out, bye-bye, and no one gets hurt. But maybe there's another alternative. Maybe it's worth a second thought. Maybe there *is* another way of seeing things, another way to live. And as she shared her personal wisdom with me, I recognized myself in her words. I, too, had a choice.

Shortly after this propitious conversation, my family and some friends decided — more on a whim than by design — to make a one-day excursion to St. Benoit du Lac, a monastic refuge in Quebec's Eastern Townships.

Someone had heard recently about a beautiful new chapel that had been added to the monastery, and we all wanted to see it. It was a one-and-a-half hour car-ride from Montreal, and as it turned out, the trip became not merely a cultural excursion, but my personal pilgrimage.

The monastery is situated on a wide expanse in the middle of the mountains. As I got out of the car, the earth firmly beneath my feet, I was struck instantly by the silence. In every direction — above, below and on either side of me — silence blanketed our surroundings. Birds flapped their wings noiselessly, whirling around the gyres; humans walked about whispering in hushed voices; and the subdued colours of nature gracefully testified to an unspeakable awe.

The moment I passed through the gates of the monastery grounds, my body became a receptacle, soaking up the serenity of the church and all creation around it. It was only much later, after I knew what meditation was, that I realized I had gone into a meditative state almost immediately. My friends were talking to me, but I didn't respond. I made no eye contact with anyone and remained still. I was taking in the silence with long, deep, exhilarating breaths. I couldn't get enough of the peace and the power that surrounded me. Everything fell into place.

On the way home, my confusion began to dissipate, and once again I was able to feel the energy of the Buddhist awareness that had attracted me in my younger years. Then it occurred to me that I should call Catherine, the mother of a friend, who had converted to Buddhism three years before. When I am ready, I thought, I will ask her to take me to the centre so that I can begin my teachings.

At my next appointment, Dr. V. was in one of his shake-her-up moods, forcing me to pause and consider the value of life, daring me to acknowledge the possibility of death. I remember exactly what he said because it was so harsh in its simplicity: "You know, Sophie, you may die." This was the first time I truly understood, in any profound sense, what was happening to me.

I replied that I was very much aware of that fact, but that I was not dead yet. I am certain I detected a tiny curvature of his lips when he realized that my words were nothing less than an indication of my progress. Later I told him about my experience at St. Benoit du Lac and my feelings about Tibet. When it is time, I said, I will find a Tibetan monk to read me the *Bardo Todol* (the Tibetan book of the dead) and help me cross over to the other side.

Wouldn't you know it, Dr. V. had participated in a conference when the Dalai Lama had visited Montreal in the early nineties, and the two of them had met. I had no doubt that this was a sign.

On my way out of his office, I decided it was time to call Catherine. I was ready. Then, all of a sudden, I had an urge to rent the movie about Tina Turner's life, *What's Love Got To Do With It?* I had always wanted to see it, but at that particular moment, I felt an impelling need. "*Now.* Sophie," I said to myself. "You go and rent that movie right now."

The movie opened with a Buddhist saying that is also a Japanese mantra. "*Nam Myoho renge kyo.*" The English translation goes something like this: "the lotus is a flower which grows in the mud. The thicker and deeper the mud, the more beautiful the flower blooms."

I decided that this was not a coincidence, either.

Within four days I received my first teachings and a short time later my meditation instructions. I started to meditate right away — forty-five minutes each morning and forty-five minutes each evening. My body and my soul were just craving it. If we count by the Gregorian calendar, my conversion may appear to have been hasty, but this was not the case. The seed of Buddhism had been planted in my teenage years, only to be cultivated in the winter of 1994.

I took Refuge (made it official) with His Eminence Tai Situ Rinpoche when he came to Montreal in January of 1995, thereby committing myself to Buddhism. The hard work with Dr. V. was also beginning to pay off, and when I entered the hospital on March 31, 1995, my mental condition was strong.

In the hospital everyone attributed my behaviour to a positive attitude. But I was not positive. I was realistic, trying my best to stay away from hope and fear. Why? Because hoping you will get better, and thus maintaining your attitude for the sole purpose of maintaining your hope, is unnatural and unhealthy. When you are in a hopeful state, you are not getting better, you are simply hoping. Grasping on to your hopes is just another way of expressing that you are scared. Hoping means you cannot accept the fact that you may die.

On the opposite end of the spectrum is fear, the constant fear that death is waiting. And what does this do to you? You cannot eat well or sleep well, you get weaker, and you are not able to tolerate your chemotherapy as well as you otherwise would.

We must all find an equilibrium between hope and fear, and live within those parameters. This balance reflects both our acceptance of death and our will to live. We are not ten years or one year away from where we are. We are now and nowhere else. There is a Tibetan saying: "tomorrow or the next life, we never know which comes first." We each have to make our own peace with our mortality, otherwise we will always be in hope and in fear. At either extreme, we are missing the point.

Once I had sorted things out, once I had come to respect myself enough to know that I had to do whatever lay in my power to survive, I became a big pain in the neck. Everything had to be my way.

One of the first things I did was refuse to wear that awful, blue hospital gown. Not because it was faded and ugly or because I always had to hide my bum, but because I didn't want to play the role of patient. I've noticed that too often we tend to act like patients. The gown is a tag, and it makes us lose our sense of individuality. I didn't want to be tagged. I was Sophie LeBlanc.

I also decided, rather early on, that I wanted to read my charts. After asking for them, however, I didn't receive an answer for over a week. It seemed no one before me had ever made such a request, and the staff didn't know what to do. As it turns out, every patient has a right to see her charts, but doctors are reluctant to permit it because they fear misinterpretation. After their initial surprise, I had no trouble seeing my charts any time I wanted, as long as it was always in the presence of a professional. I read my charts faithfully. I wanted to be on top of things, to be aware of my own case. An added benefit was that I became quite well informed concerning medical matters. Once, when I had a friend visiting and Dr. S. came to see me, my friend remarked that I knew so much about medicine I could become a doctor myself. I shook my head, looked at Dr. S., and said that I just wanted to know enough to be able to drive everyone crazy. "You're doing a great job of it," Dr. S. replied and left my room, laughing.

The information I collected from my charts came in handy on more than one occasion. I had so many infections during the course of my chemotherapy that I was often referred to the infectious-diseases physicians for the prescription of antibiotics. Once, while Dr. S. was away, we had a little run-in. They were contemplating giving me vancomycin, an antibiotic to which I was allergic. I had taken it only once, and they probably thought it was worth another try. But I was not willing to go along with this. After arguing back and forth, I told them to go to my charts where they would find a note from Dr. S. containing specific instructions that I was not to be given vancomycin under any circumstances. And that was the end of that. They had to find an alternative.

From the outset, I was determined to relate to my doctors as individuals. I can still recall one rather small and otherwise inconsequential incident involving Dr. S. As I've said, Dr. S. is a go-getter, a fighter, always running, a seemingly tireless man with a big conscience. I was going for my recreational activity one day — walking the halls of the hospital arm-in-arm with Gontrand, my IV buddy — when I noticed Dr. S. sitting at the nurses' station, an open chart in front of him, one hand holding his glasses, the other rubbing his eyes. He didn't see me approaching. "Oh, boy, are you ever exhausted," I remarked, stopping to lean on Gontrand. Dr. S. looked up at me with this big, rewarding smile on his face and said warmly, "Thank you."

My philosophy was simple. Treat your doctors as individuals, and that's exactly how they'll treat you. Treat them with respect, and they'll treat you with respect. If they don't treat you with respect, react accordingly. Soon enough, they will change their attitude.

Of course, this didn't mean that the hospital staff were my best buddies. But I do think that I managed to manoeuvre within these parameters without irking too many people. It is quite amazing what you can achieve when you allow your relationships to evolve beyond the constraints of traditional role-playing.

I'm sure it would not surprise you to learn that I was often depressed by my surroundings, and cried a lot. My remarkable head nurse, with whom I often argued and teasingly called "Mom" — which she hated — was always a significant source of support and encouragement. She would talk with me, comforting me through a crisis, riding it out with me until it had passed. She was as caring and dedicated as I could ever hope anyone to be.

On the evening preceding my daughter Natacha's first day of school, I had one of my many crises. I was very depressed because I was in the hospital receiving an intravenous antibiotic and wanted to be home with Natacha, preparing her dress and shoes and washing her hair. And I wanted to take her to school the following day. After all, this would be the first major event of her young life. When "Mom" heard about my episode, she came in to visit me. As she sat on my bed holding my hand, clearly aware of the importance of human touch during moments of debilitating despair, I suddenly had a flash. Since the intravenous antibiotic was being administered at eight-hour intervals, why couldn't she unplug me the following morning and let me out on a day-pass so that I could take Natacha to school? Whenever she could, "Mom" was always willing to accommodate me, and thought this was a great idea.

Natacha and I had a wonderful time. I felt almost normal. I waited for her until school was over — which was only about an hour — and we went to a café afterwards. It was a warm, sunny day, and I let Natacha eat as much ice-cream as she wanted. We walked for a while, hand in hand, window-shopping, talking about her teacher, and enjoying each other's company. Then I took her home, got on the metro, transferred to a bus, and walked back into the hospital in time for my medication. Natacha was happy, and I was happy. As for "Mom," she was more than happy, aware, I am sure, of the precious gift she had given me.

Seven Medical became my home, and the people there — both staff and patients — became my family. They would greet me with "Welcome home!" whenever I returned for another cycle. This was not necessarily a bad thing, for a home is a truly wonderful place. It's a place where we feel safe, where people care for each other, and where the ties are strong. At least that's what home means for me. The downside was that it made some of the deaths I witnessed that much harder to take.

Seven Medical is not the Ritz, and dying was not an extraordinary happening. During my fifth chemo cycle, I was in terrible shape. I had diarrhea. I couldn't eat. I couldn't speak. I had mouth-sores, bedsores; you name it, I had it. I couldn't read, and I wasn't even able to watch television. Time was going by drop, by drop, by drop, my IV tediously marking off the seconds. And while I was fighting for my life, I lost two dear friends.

The first was Roberto, a resident like me. We had two significant things in common. We were the same age, and we both had late-stage cancer. Whenever one of us was well enough, we would visit the other and socialize. When Roberto died, I became overwhelmed by a sense of injustice, the kind that taunts you with your own helplessness, manifesting itself as intense melancholy.

Two rooms down the hall was Giovanna. She was diagnosed while pregnant with a rare type of cancer that usually afflicts children. Giovanna and I engaged in numerous philosophical discussions, and our friendship was based on our mutual need to connect with someone in a similar circumstance, to share our feelings and, ultimately, our fears concerning the final passage from this earthly venue. At not quite full-term, labour was induced, and Giovanna died when her baby was just three months old. That was a very sad day for all of us. And when she died, I couldn't understand why it had been her instead of me. I had gone through the same thing with Roberto. Why Roberto — why not me? I could not accept the unfairness of it. My two friends had died, even though I, before being diagnosed as terminal, had harboured a strong death-wish.

There were many other times when I had difficulty keeping my emotions under control. In July I had been hooked up to an IV for several weeks because of an infection. From time to time I was unplugged in order to give my veins a rest, and on one of these occasions, I decided to get dressed and go outside for some fresh air. Not just outside the building, but outside the hospital grounds. In the streets, I became angry with every person I laid eyes on. They had their hair, and they didn't even know it. They were able to eat good food, and they didn't even know it. They were working, making love, spending time with their kids, and they didn't even know it. I wanted to scream as loudly as I could, "You are all well, and you don't even know it!"

Buddhism teaches one to acknowledge that everything is a thought. When you are angry, it is a thought. You do not welcome it; you do not banish it; you just allow it to come and go. Although it is probably difficult for non-Buddhists to understand, all feelings are thoughts. So on that hot day in July, when the world and all the people in it angered me, I allowed my anger to pass. I went to a bistro situated halfway between the hospital and down-town, sat on the open terrace, and ordered some sausages. And when I had finished, I felt better.

On my way back "home," I remembered something I had read in my philosophical days, from a book by Richard Bach. It went something like this. Question: what is a good way to find out if your mission in life is finished or not? Answer: if you are still alive, it isn't.

When I got back to the hospital, I went to the nurses' station on Seven Medical and told them I was ready. They could have my arm again.

***

February 13, 1996 was the day of my liberation. I had been in captivity for ten months, one week, and six days. It would be another month and a half before radiation started. In fact, I am undergoing radiation treatments as adjuvant therapy right now. They do my breast for six weeks, my head for four, then after a one-week respite, they radiate my spine for another two. Yet another outrageous application of elementary-school arithmetic.

I bumped into Dr. S. last week while going for coffee right after my treatments, and he asked me how the radiation was going. I told him that after what he had put me through — which I have always referred to as Hiroshima and Nagasaki with a bit of Chernobyl mixed in — radiation was like Club Med. He laughed out loud and asked me if I would mind if he used my analogy. "Just make sure it's the second part," I replied. "The first may scare people to death." He nodded in acknowledgement, then mumbled something back. I couldn't quite hear because he ran off, hurrying to another patient the way he had once hurried to me, trying, I presume, to save another life.

Afterword

One of the most important results of my spiritual healing was my acknowledgment that life involves making choices. It had been my choice, for example, to be all things to all people. It had been my choice to keep on going and going like that battery in the television commercial. It had been my choice to look after everyone but myself. And there are two main consequences to making choices. First, you are indeed in control of your life and what happens to you. Second, and much more significant, choosing also means *not* doing, *not* acting. It means letting go. It requires no effort to believe and act as if you are a victim of circumstance. It takes hard work, on the other hand, to choose to control your life by not acting, not taking on roles that require efforts of superhuman proportions, not giving in to the trappings of modern life.

Of course, certain things happen over which you have no control. I had no control over the side-effects of my treatments. But I did have control over how I would get through them. I could have sat down and cried for six months; instead, I chose to question, argue, provoke, and joke with my caregivers, to nurture my relationship with them. As a result, rather than an intimidating edifice where no one really cared, the hospital was my home.

I have taken control of all the areas of my life in which I have a choice. Now that I am, at least for the time being, in full remission, my friends are asking, what's next? What about the future? I am through the crisis, I am okay now, so they assume that everything should be back to normal. I tell them that the future for me is the end of the week. They want a ten-year plan. What about work? Work — what work? I'm *doing* my work. I am a medical experiment. In the span of almost a year, I have signed at least five research protocols. I have answered every single question that was ever asked of me, twice or even three times, by a parade of medical students and residents. I have given my body to science. I have been erased and resurrected, then erased and resurrected yet again. *This* is my work.

Admittedly, some people have a great deal of trouble with this perspective, so I tell them work has a different meaning for me now. Today, I am aware of the dangers inherent to my former world. I can recall vividly my colleagues chasing after contracts as though each assignment were a matter of life and death. And I was no different. In the communications field that is the only way to work. But nothing is a matter of life and death — after all, it was only television.

As creatures of desire, we are concerned only with those things that serve our needs, and we are interested primarily, as a result, in utility. Ego-centred beings tend to view the existence of people and objects in terms of self-gratification, not as things that are distinct and individuated, and thus valuable in their own right. Yes, I believe working is important, but in one regard only — as a contribution to the larger whole. What today's society ordinarily calls work is really something else — something centred on self, rather than others. And, for the most part, the person doing the work is the only one who gains by it.

I have also learned the value of being able to receive, that the act of accepting does not diminish my own self-worth. I have learned how to say thank you. You want to give me a ride to the hospital? Thank you. You want to take me out for lunch? Thank you, I'd love it. You want to help me clean the house? Thanks a lot.

It was while receiving my treatments that I discovered I have a tendency to extend myself beyond the limits of my physical capabilities. Knowing when to stop requires a lot of effort. I make time for myself now. In this type of life, there is room for Sophie. I do only things that satisfy me, that I enjoy. I am writing a children's book about mommies who get cancer. I volunteer with newly-diagnosed cancer patients because I believe my experience can benefit them. I have a daughter and a husband to take care of. And I study the *dharma* — the Buddhist teachings.

When Thomas Merton, with whom I began my story, talks of true prayer, we can only understand this to mean faith; faith in a Judeo-Christian context, an Asian context, a Buddhist context, or any other framework within which we lead our lives. The point is that one can achieve absolute faith, and thus a strengthening of spirit, only when there are no apparent reasons for that faith to exist. It seems that the way of the world is to cause us pain in order that we might undergo spiritual renewal. I will not attempt to answer why this is so. It *is*, and in the final analysis, that is the only thing that matters. The quest for faith and compassion is the ultimate manifestation of the human soul's capabilities.

Permit me, therefore, to leave you with this message. While I am not saying that breast cancer is a blessing, I am advocating that you seize the opportunity it provides for a personal catharsis. But first, allow yourself to have all of those reactions that result from a sudden threat to your mortality. It is natural to experience pain and anger and helplessness. Go through them, then let them pass. They will.

And know that these experiences will, in time, reveal the person that you truly are — a genuine human being, compassionate both toward yourself and toward others. Humankind deserves your goodness, and you deserve the goodness of others.

[Author's note: Sadly, Sophie LeBlanc's life and work ended with her passing in the winter of 1998 as we were finishing this book. Her children's book, A Dragon in Your Head, *was published by Publications MNH in October 1997. She is missed by everyone who knew her.]*

Hema Dias Abeygunawardena

Toronto, Ontario
Date of birth: June 21, 1942
Date of diagnosis: April 1991

I had been living in Canada less than a year when my youngest son, Vikum, called me to the window, excited. "Mama, Mama, come and see the racoon!" The racoon was not the only reason for Vikum's excitement that day. In the afternoon his father had finally arrived, after being separated from us for ten long months.

I went to the window where my son was standing, and together we watched the racoon foraging in our new backyard. My husband, Hector, was in the bedroom, sleeping off the long drive that had brought him from Massachusetts to Toronto. The landlady with whom we were sharing the house was having tea and cakes in the kitchen. And, for no reason at all, my hand went to my breast. Could this be cancer? Motionless, I stood by the window, unable to share in my young son's happiness.

In the days that followed, I was overcome by the fear of having to face a disease I knew little about, in a host-culture that was still unfamiliar to me.

Had I been at home, in Sri Lanka, my husband and my brothers would have joined forces immediately to find me the best doctor and the best available treatment in the country. I would have gone to the hospital with my sisters, and my nieces would have cared for my children. My sole responsibility would have been to concentrate on getting well.

Instead, I found myself alone with a ten-year-old and a newly arrived husband, facing the first crisis of my life without my family's help.

***

I was born in Sri Lanka (Ceylon at the time), in the southern province of Galle, on June 21, 1942. It was the Riviera of South Asia then, a thriving and beautiful country still under British rule. My identical twin sister and I, the last of nine children, were separated soon after our birth. My mother was unable to feed yet another two mouths, so my sister was adopted by my uncle and his wife. I was spared, and got to grow up with seven other siblings and my parents.

In many respects, our house was a self-contained community where life was defined by human connections. And I learned how to share more than just food, shelter, and clothing, although these too were issues. I still have memories of my mother cutting a mango into ten equal pieces — in awe of her ability to apportion everything into ten — and then putting a slice away for my eldest brother, who wouldn't be home from work until after dark. I wanted to eat that slice so badly, but mother said I could have it only if my brother offered it to me. I waited and waited for him to get home, one eye on the saucer containing the mango — we had no refrigerator — the other eye on our front door.

In spite of all the age differences, our family was very close, and we were strongly committed to one another. We grew up without shame in asking for each other's help, and it was natural for me to rely on my family whenever I needed them. So on that beautiful early evening in the spring of 1991, I discovered more than the lump in my breast. I discovered solitude.

***

It had been chance really, a series of unforeseen circumstances, that had brought us first out of Sri Lanka and eventually to Canada.

I was only seventeen when I met and fell in love with Hector. But I knew from the start that being a devoted wife, to the exclusion of everything else, would not be an entirely fulfilling life for me. In Sri Lanka, education is highly valued and we have a very high literacy rate among men and women alike. I went to university and became a teacher. Then, when I was twenty-four, I married Hector, who had also completed his teaching certificate, and we both started our professional lives in a remote area away from our home town.

Within two years our first son, Vish, was born, and six years later our second son, Vinodh, arrived. In time, Hector became vice-principal of the school, and we made a comfortable living. I continued to teach, but in order to qualify for annual wage increases, I needed a Diploma in Education in addition to my BA degree. One day the idea came to me to go back to school, and even though this meant that as a family we would be separated, Hector supported my decision. Our elder son, Vish, was already away from home, boarding at the Royal College on a scholarship. I would attend university in the capital city, Colombo, two hundred kilometres from where we were living in Welimada, Nuwara Eliya district.

Hector and I agreed that I should take our three-year-old son with me, and so the two of us went away to Colombo to live with my brother and his family. That year was very special for us both: while Vinodh was pampered by his cousins, I had time to concentrate on my studies.

Having graduated with a merit pass, I was selected to enroll in the Master's programme in the faculty of Education. This time, however, Hector didn't want me to continue. He said that there had been enough disruption in our lives, and his disapproval presented a big dilemma for me. Half of me wanted to go on with my studies; the other half wanted to please my husband. In the end, I recognized that Hector was right and rejected the university's offer.

A few weeks later we received a letter from the Dean, addressed to my husband, requesting that we both attend a meeting with him in his office. The Dean was one of Hector's former teachers, and in our culture, one does not say "no" to a person of higher status. He greeted us in a professorial tone, befitting his position — "Are you people thinking clearly?" — and after an hour of pleasant conversation, I heard my husband say, "Certainly, Hema will enroll." There were handshakes and smiles all around.

By the time I completed all the requirements of the Master's programme, Hector and I had three sons, and we had moved permanently to Colombo, which meant that Hector had to commute to his job in Nuwara Eliya. Nonetheless, it was a joy to have our family together again. The boys were growing, all doing well in school, Hector was happy in his new position as an Education officer, and after a short return to teaching, I decided that my goals could be better achieved working at the Ministry of Education.

In 1985, mostly at the urging of my eldest son, I applied for a Fulbright scholarship for study in the United States. Of course, it was to my great advantage that I had written my Master's thesis in English, something my academic advisor had suggested and, in fact, had taken all the way to the university's senate on my behalf. By that time in our history, language was a big political issue. After Sri Lanka gained independence from Great Britain, nationalist sentiment penetrated all aspects of life, and the two native languages — Tamil and Sinhalese — predominated, especially in academia. I was very fortunate that my advisor had such foresight, as well as genuine concern for her students.

I was awarded the Fulbright scholarship, and we left for the University of Massachusetts in the fall of 1986 for what was to be a one-year stay. Hector had arranged a leave of absence from his job, and our third son, Vikum, came with us. The two elder boys stayed at home to continue their schooling, and were looked after well by both our families. Shortly after we left Sri Lanka, however, the conflict between Sinhalese Buddhists and Tamil Hindus erupted nation-wide, and the country was thrown into turmoil. Clearly, our best option was to prolong our stay in America. I applied for a tuition-waver at the University of Massachusetts and enrolled in the Doctorate programme. We brought out our two other sons, and Hector got a job at the university library.

We lived in America for four and a half years. Then in 1990, I had a chance meeting with some professors from OISE (The Ontario Institute for Studies in Education), who invited me to continue my studies there. OISE is well-known and has an excellent reputation back home. Also, we thought that Canada, as a member of the Commonwealth, would make a better host-culture for us than the United States. I left for Toronto with ten-year-old Vikum, while Hector stayed in Massachusetts until our middle son finished high school. Vish, the eldest, had one year left at university and had been selected to go to Japan for an internship in economics upon completion of his degree.

Ten months after Vikum and I left the States for Canada, Vinodh had finished high school, Vish was on his way to Japan, and Hector would soon join us. I anticipated our reunion with great joy and spent many hours preparing my husband's favourite meals. Vikum was very excited the day his father arrived. Exhausted from his trip, Hector embraced us both and went directly to sleep. And Vikum called me to the window to look at the racoon.

For two long weeks I kept the lump in my breast a secret, trying to buy time, convincing myself that it couldn't be malignant. After all, I was full of energy and had no symptoms of disease. And surely breast cancer was a western woman's disease. Most important of all, as a Buddhist, I didn't believe that my consciousness had created any bad karma in a previous birth for which I would now have to suffer.

But when I finally decided to tell my husband about it, he insisted right away that I go to the doctor. What doctor, I asked him. He didn't know, and neither did I. We were unfamiliar with the Canadian healthcare system.

Hector asked me every day what I planned to do about my situation. To stop his nagging, I promised I would go to the health clinic at the university. However, on the day of my appointment, I walked across the campus, hesitating all the way, before finally stopping on the front steps of the building and turning back. Three times I made an appointment, and three times I left without going inside. After my last attempt, Hector said to me, "Hema, if you don't go to the doctor, I'm not going to talk to you." He was very serious, but I started to laugh. "Oh, I think I can live with that," I answered. (Hector never carried out his threat.)

It must have been the discipline of my Buddhist upbringing that led me eventually to the library. I spent hours reading up on breast cancer, study after study, but this turned out to be a very disappointing experience. One report said one thing, another something else. And the more I read, the more confused I became. Much of the information was contradictory. However, one good thing did result from my efforts. I became more objective about my situation, enough to realize that pretending I wasn't sick didn't make it so.

Thinking that she would be the best person to confide in, I approached a research colleague at the university who was also a nurse at Sunnybrook hospital. Immediately, Diana put herself in charge. First, she made a point of requesting that I see a female doctor at the health clinic, and for this I was very grateful, as well as surprised, because the issue had never come up in our discussions. Later, she made the cross-campus walk to the building with me, holding on to my arm to make sure I wouldn't turn back again. She took me for my mammogram, my first visit to the surgeon, and even to the hospital for my biopsy. With Diana by my side, I felt very safe. It wasn't that I didn't want my husband there, but Hector had been in Canada less than a month, and was not equipped to help me at this stage.

Three days after my biopsy, Hector and I went to the American embassy to get our visas for the States. We desperately wanted to be with our middle son, Vinodh, at his high school graduation ceremony. When we arrived home from the embassy, however, there was a message on the answering machine from the surgeon.

In less than an hour we were sitting in his office listening to my cancer diagnosis. I was told that I would probably need a mastectomy because the lump was quite large — three and a half centimetres — and very close to my chest wall. The doctor would arrange for me to get a hospital bed right away. I remember that he was holding my open file in his hands as he spoke, and for some reason that image scared me more than what he was saying. Even today I can still see that open folder with my name on it. I didn't want to know any details. I didn't ask any probing questions. The only thing I wanted to do was leave. I felt myself going deeper and deeper into the other side — into death — and I had to get out of there. I told the surgeon that I was sorry, but I wouldn't be able to make it. We had to attend our son's graduation in the States. With that, I left his office.

Hector must have sensed what I was thinking because on our way home he said to me, "Hema, I'm not worried. I'm sure you believe the worst but I don't believe I'm unlucky enough to lose you." I was feeling sorry for him, imagining the hardships he would face without me, but that was not in Hector's thoughts. He didn't throw self-pity at me, saying, "Oh, dear, what will I do when you are sick?" Instead, he talked about all the problems we had solved together as husband and wife. This would be just one more to get through.

We left for the States the following morning, and the moment we crossed the border I was thinking, "I'll be okay here. I am safe. I'm across the border now." I know that sounds crazy. I suppose what I really felt was the healing power of familiar surroundings and faces. And there was one other thing. Massachusetts has a very special temple called the Peace Pagoda, and it was with great promise that I anticipated going there.

After Vinodh's graduation — a very proud event for all of us — we made the trip to the Peace Pagoda to request that the nuns pray for me. In their rituals for sick people, the nuns beat the drum in a special way to get rid of all the negative elements surrounding the body. It was an intense and solemn spiritual experience, and when we made our departure, I was at peace, ready to accept my future. My confidence was restored.

We stayed in the States for two more days, visiting with friends, eating out, and partying. All I wanted to do was have fun. Perhaps in the back of my mind I was thinking that I'd better have a little happiness before I die.

The idea that it was time to act gradually took hold of me during our return trip to Canada. But first, I had to tell my academic advisor at OISE that I would be unable to finish my papers on time. By then it was early May and the semester was almost over. I was so nervous and shy that I had no idea how to go about it or what to say. And my advisor was a man, which only made things worse.

Eventually, I decided that the easiest way to handle this would be by e-mail. My advisor replied, telling me how sorry he was, and asked me to call a certain professor in my department. I couldn't understand why he wanted me to do this. I had taken only one course with her, and we didn't know each other well.

As a student I was reluctant to approach her. Then *she* called me! It turned out that she had had breast cancer too, and when she told me about her experience I was very humbled. Like me, she had found it difficult to confront her own denial. "You must grieve and you must cry," she said, "instead of waiting for a miracle to happen." I felt as if she were reading my thoughts, and I bonded with her instantly. All breast cancer survivors are equals; I know that today.

A big weight was lifted from my shoulders now that I finally felt connected with someone. In truth, I had been looking for my courage, hoping to find it through others. I began to talk about my situation openly, at least among my university associates. And to my surprise, I received a message from another professor, Marlene. I was excited and honoured when she said she wanted to see me.

Marlene is the warmest and smartest woman I have ever known. She is the head of the Centre for Applied Cognitive Science, a very important position. I sat in her office for one and a half hours — the office of a high-ranking professor! — full of self-pity and pain. I may have said it out loud, I'm not sure, but I was overwhelmed by the question I couldn't answer. Why was this happening to me? Marlene was sitting behind her desk, and I was in a chair in front of her. At one point she said to me, "Hema, you're a Buddhist, and I know what you are thinking. You're thinking that this is a punishment because you have not been perfect in some other life." I nodded. Then she got up from her chair and came very close to me. She placed her hands on my shoulders, bent down so that she was level with my face, and stared into my eyes. She looked as if she were about to reveal a big secret. She whispered,

"Hema, are you perfect in *this* life?" I burst out laughing. "No," I replied. "Well, you're going to work off your bad karma in a very positive way," she said. "Sunnybrook is a good hospital, and they know what they are doing." Then, she went on to say that if I ever needed her support, financial or otherwise, she would be there for me. I had no doubt Marlene was speaking the truth.

The next morning I called the surgeon to tell him I was ready, but first I felt I had to apologize for my previous behaviour. Doctors command the highest respect in our culture, and dismissing a doctor the way I had done is considered very rude. However, my apologies didn't matter to him; he was simply relieved that I had finally decided to get treatment.

On the eve of my surgery, in spite of what that first female professor had told me, there *was* a miracle. It wasn't exactly what I had hoped for, but for a miracle it was close enough. This is what happened.

In Sri Lanka, before an operation, you must go to the temple to perform certain rituals, similar to what the nuns had done for me at the Peace Pagoda. Your entire family, your friends, and everyone who knows and cares about you participates, to evoke the blessings that will neutralize the negative forces around you.

I had no one to do this for me. No one in Canada and, especially, no one at home. This was because I had been very particular about who should and shouldn't know about my condition. And I had had good reasons for all of my choices. For example, one family with whom we had become very good friends was expecting a baby, and one does not give bad news to a pregnant woman. A mother must always be happy while her child is inside her. As for confiding in other people from my community, to be totally honest, I didn't want them looking at me, thinking, "Poor Hema. What a pity."

I also didn't tell my brothers and sisters and Hector's family back home. There was no point in having them worry. They were so far away that there was nothing practical they could do for me. I intended to call them only after the operation.

I had kept it from Vikum, but the two older boys knew. If I am going to die, I thought, my sons should have an opportunity to say goodbye to me in whatever manner they choose.

Now here is the important thing. On his way to Japan, Vish had stopped off in the Phillippines for a three-week seminar related to his Japanese internship. But when he went to get his visa from the Japanese embassy he was told that he had to go home, to his country of origin, and apply for a visa from there. Vish arrived in Colombo the day before my operation, and *he* became my messenger. With a difference of ten hours between us, he had enough time to tell all my brothers and sisters and my husband's family about me. That same night everyone went to the temple to offer *pujas* for my speedy recovery. As for Vish, he performed the rituals to his heart's content. Who else but a son should evoke blessings for his mother! Just as it is written.

On the eve of my surgery, when Hector told me what had taken place just a few hours before, I had no doubt I would make it.

This was the first miracle, from my first son. The second miracle came from my second son.

I was under the impression that the surgery alone would fully treat my breast cancer. At most I expected to get radiation. But when malignancy was found in my lymph nodes, I was told I would also need six months of intensive chemotherapy.

At my first session with the oncologist, I was given a four-page document listing all of its potential side-effects. This frightened me so much that I decided not to take the treatments. After a couple of weeks, however, I became very agitated. What if the cancer came back! Every time I looked at Vikum, I became more scared. I had fulfilled my duty toward my two older sons, but Vikum needed to be looked after for a few more years. So I changed my mind and began the chemo. Physically, it was the most horrible experience of my life.

And my hair! In Sri Lanka, long hair is one of the most celebrated aspects of beauty, and when I was growing up I wore my hair long all the time. By the second month of my treatments, I was completely bald. My hair fell out as if it had been previously pasted onto my scalp. I couldn't even look in the mirror in the morning until I had put on a wig or a scarf.

It never ever occurred to me that my hair would grow back. I associated a lack of hair with old age, and mine had started to thin out even before my health problems. So I assumed that the chemotherapy had only hastened what was the normal course of nature, and I expected to be bald for the rest of my life. Even when that professor, my first breast cancer soul-mate, told me that her hair had grown back, I attributed it to her unique genetic make-up. She was from the Middle East, and I didn't think her situation applied to me.

Of my whole cancer experience, losing my hair was the worst, more traumatic than losing my breast. The breast is concealed, and if I didn't say anything you would never know I'd lost it. But hair is an altogether different matter.

And so, there I was, not only feeling very ill but also feeling ugly. I think that most of the side-effects I had read about eventually manifested themselves in my body. My husband, who had a job by then (he was working as a security officer), changed his shift so that either he or Vikum would always be home with me. At that stage, of course, it was impossible to hide my illness from Vikum, and I realized that it had been a big mistake to do so in the first place.

On the weekends, people from my community would come over, and that was really terrible. No one knew how to react. They'd ask, "Hema, how are you?" and I would reply that I was fine. This would be followed by silence. They didn't know what to say next, and it seemed they all expected *me* to continue. After a while I told my husband, "I can't deal with these people. I can't. I can't."

I was so sick that I wanted to die. I closed my eyes and waited, but nothing happened. I tried it again, and again nothing happened. After several failed attempts, I realized that one cannot force death to come. Death comes in its own time. Therefore, I thought, I must still have something to live for.

At two o'clock in the afternoon, on a particularly difficult day when I was still in my nightdress, I began to focus on a sign, a miracle, to show me my true purpose in life. I concentrated harder and harder but I was not successful. I went to the kitchen to make myself a cup of tea, to drown my confused thoughts, when I heard a knock at the kitchen door. It was my middle son, Vinodh. I had not seen him since his high school graduation, some six months ago, and I couldn't believe my eyes.

Vinodh had remained in the States after Hector came to Canada, and he was now a first-year student at the Rochester Institute of Technology. He and a friend had rented a car from the university the previous day — four days of unlimited mileage for $99 U.S. They drove to Toronto, and when they couldn't find Charles Street in the dark, they turned around and went back to New York. At dawn the next morning, they set out again, taking turns sleeping in the back seat. They arrived shortly after two in the afternoon when I was in the kitchen making tea.

Vinodh's appearance within minutes of my asking for a miracle confirmed for me that *he* was the miracle. I knew that my work on earth had not yet been fulfilled. I still had things to do for my sons — especially for Vikum, my youngest, which meant giving him the opportunity to take care of me. Vikum knew that his father was relying on him, as were his brothers, who could not be present to share the load. This was a huge responsibility for a small child, and as a result, Vikum has grown up to be my "loving proof" — a compassionate and caring young man.

***

Chemotherapy ended in March of 1992, and radiation three weeks later. Then everything was over. Hector said to me, "Hema, put all your cancer books away. Now you are back to normal." But it never became normal. Something had changed.

Once I had gained distance from the drama of the past eight months, I was able to reflect upon it more objectively. I realized that my biggest problem had been that I hadn't known even one Sinhalese woman with breast cancer. The trouble is that women from my community keep quiet about this disease. In Sri Lanka, a few years ago, I had a cousin who died of breast cancer. She didn't want to go for treatment, and no one talked about her illness. When she died no one knew why. And in India, when a woman dies of breast cancer, her death certificate states that she died of natural causes.

Immigrant women come to this country carrying their customs with them. A friend, who is also a survivor, recently told me how lucky I am to have sons, because this allows me to talk freely about my disease. She could never do that, she said. She has two daughters, and she is afraid that if people find out about her illness, the girls will have trouble getting married. She may be right in her own way, but I disagree with that philosophy. I wouldn't mind if one of my sons married a woman whose mother had had breast cancer. (Now that would be a real treat! Two mothers-in-law with breast cancer.)

For me it was easy to come out of the closet, and it had nothing to do with the gender of my children. It was a natural continuation of the work I had begun at home — fighting for women's rights and drawing attention to women's issues. As a result, I changed the direction of my Ph.D. research and I am now concentrating on how immigrant families communicate on health issues.

Also, I've become a breast cancer spokesperson in the immigrant community. We need to have gentle persuasion to change old attitudes and beliefs. It is not easy; it takes time to get used to a new culture. I try to make immigrant women aware that breast cancer can happen to them. When we are living in a host-culture, we don't cook the same way, we don't have the same rituals or the same lifestyles that we had back home. I can't remember the last time I sat down with my whole family for dinner on a weekday. At home we always ate together. In the modern, western world, with all its noise, distractions, and different work-patterns, we have lost our quiet times and the ability to be with ourselves first. Our heritage does not exempt us from western diseases.

Immigrant women must realize that they have to go for regular check-ups. They need to know what to do after they are diagnosed. They have to learn that hiding their disease is wrong. And they must talk about their feelings.

I remember my very first visit with a Sinhalese woman the day after her breast surgery. The first thing I said to her was, "This is my real hair. Just pull on it and you'll see." I knew this would make her feel better, and it was also good for breaking the ice. From then on, she felt safe with me and was more open about her feelings. Some time later, after she was through the worst, she told me that the day she had seen me walking and talking was the day her life changed.

I am also involved with an outreach programme whose members visit various cultural groups. Not long ago I participated in a native ceremony called the "healing circle." When I talked about my life, I related a specific conversation I'd had with each of my three sons. It went something like this: Should I ever become unconscious, I told them, I still wanted them to come to see me. To nurse me, talk to me, touch me, change my sheets, take care of me. Because I am their mother.

As soon as I had finished, a man sitting across from me suddenly began to cry. Recounting the circumstances of his own mother's death, he explained that when she lay dying, she had been surrounded by a large group of women who were caring for her, and that he hadn't known what to do. Had he heard my talk before, he said, he would have barged right through those women to hold his mother's hand.

This was a very bittersweet moment in my life. I understood the man's pain, and at the same time it confirmed for me that I was doing something of value.

Afterword

Growing up, I didn't always pay attention to my mother. In fact, it was only after my breast cancer, at the age of forty-nine, that I was able to understand what she was trying to teach us. In her own special way, she was a philosopher. Anyone would have to be with eight children in the house. One of the things she used to say was this: "If you have lemons, make lemonade. But just squeezing them won't do. You have to add some water, some sugar, some salt. And don't put in too much salt simply because it's cheap."

Of all the lessons in this message, one in particular affected me more than the rest — that you can't do it alone. You can squeeze yourself as much as your strength allows, but you need help from others to live a full and varied life.

Here's just one example. During my entire married life, it was I who had ruled the kitchen. I was the one who decided when to go shopping, what to eat, or whom we would invite for dinner. The kitchen had been my domain. When I got sick from the chemo and wasn't able to cook, it was a great shock for me to see Hector and Vikum enjoying a plate of spaghetti that Hector had prepared. Now Hector is an expert in making rice and curry, and also coffee.

Breast cancer has robbed me of my biggest power, but I haven't tried to take it back. Today everyone participates in the kitchen. And when guests want to know the ingredients of a certain dish, I am proud to tell them to ask my husband or one of my sons. Other things validate me now, such as taking the message of breast-health to various communities, or helping people who are living with this illness.

My mother couldn't have prepared me for breast cancer. Instead, she tried to prepare me for life. I am minus one breast, but I am also more than the sum of my body parts. And, remembering my mother's wisdom, I try to make every day of my life a lemonade.

One last thing: in my next birth, I plan to get my Ph.D. when I'm sixteen, not fifty-six.

Brenda Williamson

Toronto, Ontario
Date of birth: June 1, 1950
Date of diagnosis: Spring, 1988

When asked to consider participating in this anthology of breast cancer survivors, I was hesitant at first. What do I have to say that could benefit other women? I do not have a recipe to share; I cannot provide a fast and ready guide; I don't even have a list of do's and don't's for how one should manage such an unparalleled crisis. Furthermore, although I've never gone out of my way to hide my illness, like most Black women I have certainly not been public about it.

However, I did realize immediately that, if nothing else, because I am still alive, I could perhaps save others the type of anguish that I have had to bear.

After my operation, once I had quieted down a little, I began searching for a role model to fashion my life after. Doing what someone else was doing to fight her disease would, I thought, guarantee me the same successful outcome. Jill Ireland was one of the few celebrities who had gone public with her illness at the time, so I chose her. I read her book and then anxiously kept tabs on her condition. Heartened by her progress in the face of multiple recurrences, I felt confident that I, too, would come out of this alive. Then, tragically, Jill Ireland succumbed to her disease, and I was left utterly devastated, convinced that I'd be next in line.

Thankfully, by the grace of God, I wasn't. Ten years later I'm still here. I'm healthy and happy. And although I would never put myself up as a role model for anyone, the opportunity to let others know that I survived was something that I could not, in good conscience, pass up.

So, I began to think about the shape my story would take, reflecting on my many years of living with breast cancer. In the process, I often found myself facing some deeply personal issues for the very first time, creating in me a new level of awareness about myself, about life, about this disease. I recognized that embarking on a journey of self-discovery is a unique, individual matter, often dictated by circumstance. There are women who begin this journey the moment they are diagnosed. Some wait until the end of their treatments. Still others may never embark on it. In any case, even if we delay this journey — as I did for ten years — or never make it at all, we need not admonish ourselves. Dealing with breast cancer is difficult enough, without feeling we have to find a profound, spiritual meaning behind it.

I also believe that it is perfectly okay for us to resume normal lives. Personally, I have not made major life-altering decisions as a result of my illness. I did not have an epiphany of any kind; my perception of the world did not change. I have become no more religious than before and have turned neither into a feminist nor an activist. To the extent that we are heroes — and I'm not saying necessarily that we are — our heroism is not derived from acts that make the talk-show circuit, that appear heroic to the general public. Last year I read about a group of breast cancer survivors who had challenged themselves to a gruelling survival-training programme called "outward bound." This is fine for women who want to do such things, breast cancer or no breast cancer. But our true heroism is silent and invisible. It lies in the daily battles we wage, emotionally and physically, to combat this ever-present threat to our lives. I had a wonderful life before breast cancer and am not ashamed to admit that I wanted to keep it that way.

Sometimes it is a waste to leave happy endings for the end, so I will begin my story there, with who I am today, and how I feel at this point in my life.

***

I have an exciting, public relations job that I've held for the past twenty years, working for a non-profit organization that publicizes and encourages the use of steel. Just the other day I participated in a four-day education seminar, here in Toronto, that brought together engineering professors from across the country. One of our activities included a tour of the construction site of the new Air Canada Raptor's arena, not to be recorded as one of the most pleasant experiences I've ever had. It was bitterly cold — one of those February days when the wind blows through your skin right into your bones — and the higher we went the windier it became. But this is Canada after all, and I have no reason to complain. Canada is my adopted country, wind, hail and ice-storms included.

It was not by chance that I chose a career in which physical decorum is essential. Taking pride in my appearance is something that my mother drilled into me, as she did into all her children, early in life. By the age of five I had a little nylon hat, a matching pair of gloves, and several pretty dresses from which to choose to go to church and Sunday school. Every Sunday, three rows of Williamson's — there were seven of us, including my parents — would walk across the town in our starched and perfectly pressed outfits, mother in back keeping a strict eye on the wannabe-motley crew in front of her. If ever she spied a stooped shoulder, a bent back, or a similarly offensive act, she'd approach the culprit stealthily, bending down to whisper, "Keep your back straight, get that chin up," before casually falling back to take my father's arm and resume her weekly exchange with the neighbours. When I became a mother myself, I, too, tried to set a good example for my three daughters, aiming to instil in them dignity of body and mind. In addition, I was the type of person who never allowed a single strand of hair to be out of place. If I chipped a nail and had no emery-board handy, I considered it nothing short of a disaster. Then I lost a breast and learned the true meaning of impairment.

But all this happened a long time ago, and today my feelings about the integrity of my body are not as strong as they once were. Whether this is due to the fact that I eventually underwent breast reconstruction, or simply that I'm ten years older and what is important to me has changed, I don't really know. The truth is I don't think about it much.

In my personal life I have Roy, my husband of almost twenty years. Our three daughters are away at college, and not having to worry any more about their comings and goings has greatly diminished my daily stress. I love my children dearly, but as any parent with daughters of dating age can appreciate, pacing the floor when one of the girls is an hour past her curfew is not something I will ever miss.

Last year — I don't know why — I got it into my head that Roy and I should become foster-parents. We have the means to support another child, and goodness knows there are too many kids these days in need of a stable home-environment. The idea fell by the wayside, however, when my middle daughter, Tambudzai, said to me, "Mama, are you crazy? I thought you would have learned by now that taking on the problems of the world is not good for your health." She had a point. With breast cancer one is never completely out of the woods. And when I found out that I needed a medical certificate to qualify as a foster-parent, I knew that my doctor would try to talk me out of it. So where does all this leave me now? I have a luxury that I've never had before — time to concentrate on myself and do whatever I enjoy. Painting, perhaps. That's something I've always wanted to try. To tell you the truth, I am not in a hurry to commit to anything. After a full day's work, it is very seductive to come home to a comfortable house with every conceivable amenity, get into the Jacuzzi, read, watch television, or just relax with Roy.

I think I have now arrived at the chronological beginning of my story, in Jamaica, where I started life forty-eight years ago.

***

I was born in a rural parish, in my great-grandparents' home, the third of five children. It was a huge plantation-type house, old and in need of repair, but it had many rooms and many people lived there — my parents, my older brother and sister, my great-grandparents, and one uncle with his family. We didn't have much in terms of modern conveniences, things like running water, indoor plumbing, or even a telephone, but hardship was a way of life and the only life I knew. I was a cheerful little girl and never really missed anything, content with all the love around me, learning of nothing but the goodness of the world.

When my fifth and last sibling arrived, even that big old house became too cramped, and my parents decided to move to a smaller home, one that would be ours alone.

In the years following the war, Great Britain welcomed immigrants from the colonies (Jamaica gained independence in 1962), and my father was enticed by the prospect of creating a better life for his family. Because he had never felt any hostility toward the British — in fact, he had joined the RAF during the war — when the opportunity came, he left for England. My mother followed him in 1960, and we, the children, went to live with our great-aunt, Vena. Aunt Vena was very much like our mother — although she came from our father's side of the family — religious, strict, and generous at heart, but she had no children of her own. As if five were not enough for her to handle, she opened her home to needy kids from other parishes, and at one time, as many as ten of us were living with her. It was while we waited to go to England — which would not be for another four years — that I developed an overwhelming sense of responsibility for my two smaller sisters. I don't really know how this urge came about. They were only two and three years younger than me, the other kids in the house never bothered us, and Aunt Vena filled our mother's shoes to a tee. Nonetheless, I considered myself the protector of my family's welfare and, from then on, became the person in charge, the one who'd fix everyone's problems.

We made the journey to England in 1964 and were finally reunited with our parents. England meant Somerset, more specifically, the city of Bath, which I grew to appreciate as the most gorgeous place on earth only after I had left it. Bath is famous for its hot springs, of course, but nature has blessed it in other ways, from the rounded hills that surround the city to deep underground caves with magical, multicoloured stalactites. It is a quaint, old city of tight, winding streets, few open spaces, and many forms of twentieth-century construction cramped alongside historic Georgian architecture.

As a fourteen-year-old, all this beauty was lost on me, but as a Black youngster coming from a relatively poor country, I was quickly attracted by what I perceived to be limitless opportunities for creating a comfortable life. I saw by my parents' example that if you worked hard, you reaped the rewards. We lived in a spacious corner townhouse, whose depth and height more than made up for its conventional British narrowness. There was a large garden at the back where my father spent his time cultivating his rose-bushes — the prettiest on the street, I might add. And we had a car, more for travelling the countryside than commuting.

At nineteen, attracted by the glitz, the glamour, and the lights, I left for London and moved in with my elder sister, who had a flat there. When a friend from Toronto invited me over for a visit, my adventurous side jumped at the chance. Of all the countries in the Commonwealth, Canada had always been the most mysterious to me. I was intrigued not only by the concept of shivering cold, but also by the people — modern, like I had become — who chose to take it all in stride.

I had money saved to pay for a three-week vacation and arrived in Canada at the end of September, 1971, to what was an extraordinary Indian summer. In the third week of my visit I chanced on an interesting job with the Toronto Zoological Society, and said to myself, why not? I wouldn't mind staying here awhile. Then I met my future husband and committed myself not only to marriage, but also to Canada. It was with the latter that I had a true love affair; the marriage was a disaster.

Four years later, I began life as a twenty-six-year-old single mother with two small children and a fate prescribed by conventional wisdom. Doomed to be just another statistic, I'd be alone and poor for the rest of my life. Even I began to think that no man would be interested in me, given that I was part of a larger package. But I was lucky enough to defy the odds, and six months after my divorce I met Roy. Had I gone to a dating service with a comprehensive wish-list in hand, I couldn't have found a more perfect partner. We were married and began a life of devotion, hard work, and success. Our third daughter was born in 1978.

There was only one thing wrong with our Canadian dream. I had left my parents and siblings permanently behind.

***

In 1987 breast cancer awareness was not as widespread as it is today, so when I went to my doctor to tell him about a small lump in my breast, his reaction didn't offend me. Okay, I thought, he knows best, so "we'll watch it." A few months later I discovered a concentration of lumps, some distance away from the original, but my doctor couldn't feel anything.

Later that year I was vacationing with one of my sisters, who had become a nurse, and when I told her that the cluster of lumps seemed to be getting larger, she immediately admonished me to have it checked out. I came home and my doctor arranged for a mammogram. After the results were in, he said that he wanted to do a needle aspiration, just to be on the safe side.

My initial reaction was no. Maybe I was scared of that huge needle, or maybe I was so frightened that I just wanted to gain a reprieve from the catastrophe lurking in the back of my mind. And without pursuing the matter further — he didn't even ask me twice — my doctor simply raised his eyebrows and gave in. I went home, and that was the end of that. I still shiver when I recall that this actually happened.

A few months passed and I decided to see him again, because it felt as if the lumps were growing. At this point he sent me to a specialist. Tauja, my ten-year-old, didn't have school that day, and she wanted to accompany me. I had told the girls about the possibility of cancer, so Tauja knew why we were going to the doctor.

I left her in the waiting room as I disappeared behind closed doors, listening to the surgeon tell me that I would have to be hospitalized right away. He said that he was quite certain about a malignancy, but only a surgical biopsy would yield a definitive diagnosis. If, indeed, the lumps turned out to be cancerous, he said, he would remove my breast right on the spot. Oh my goodness, I remember thinking, this all seems a little drastic. I told him I'd go home and think about it.

On our way out, Tauja began fidgeting and in a hushed voice asked, "What did he say, Mama? What did he say?" I began to tell her, but as we got into an elevator full of people, Tauja put her index finger to her lips and said, "Later, Mama." Clearly inhibited by the strangers who were intruding on our privacy, she was worried about being overheard.

All the way down I was asking myself, how do I tell her? *What* do I tell her? That her Mama is going to lose a breast? That her Mama is going to die? I think the hardest part of dealing with this disease has always been protecting my loved ones from their personal pain. I had the strength to protect them from *my* pain; I could control *my* emotions. But I had no power over free-falling imaginations. It was in the elevator that I realized the wicked irony of a mother's obligation. Throughout our lives we try to protect our children from harm, but in the final analysis, we cannot protect them from the worst harm of all — our own demise.

Tauja and I arrived on the ground floor, moved a few feet away to a place where we'd be alone and, using a matter-of-fact tone, I told her that the doctor might want to remove my breast. I also told her that I would never agree to something like that. Tauja seemed relieved by my determination, as if my refusal were some kind of evidence that the situation was not as serious as she had envisioned.

Later that night I kept mostly to myself, while Roy took care of the girls. I wasn't ready to go into the hospital and wake up with only one breast on my body. That much I knew. And I remembered having heard recently about a new surgical procedure called a partial mastectomy. Not knowing better, that was what I decided I wanted.

This time, with Roy by my side, I returned to my own doctor and explained how distressed I had become after my visit with the specialist. The doctor then offered to refer me to another, "more conservative" surgeon. He turned out to be an older gentleman, much more sympathetic than the first, and although he told us essentially the same thing, there was one big difference. He'd allow a week between the biopsy and the surgery to give me a chance to prepare emotionally for the shock of losing a breast. I felt much more comfortable with this scenario. But what foolishness on my part! One can never be adequately prepared for such a thing.

Within a week, and one year after having gone to the doctor with my problem, I lay on a gurney, covered by a faded hospital gown and a bleached-thin blanket, furtively attempting to touch my breast in the last moments of its existence. A few days later, news came that four of my lymph nodes contained cancer cells, and the decision was made to put me on chemotherapy.

This was an unexpected turn of events — all along I had thought everything would be taken care of with the surgery — and what terrified me more than anything was the prospect of losing my hair. I had already lost a breast. I could never, ever get used to being bald.

I was told that hair-loss would not necessarily occur with the particular drugs I'd be given, a combination known as CMF, but I wasn't going to leave anything to chance. My sister reminded me of my mother's saying, "a woman's beauty is in her hair." So, before my treatments began, I decided to get it braided. It took my hairdresser four painstaking hours, working on only a few strands at a time, to create something in the order of a hundred separate braids. Then, for the duration of my chemotherapy, I never touched my hair again. I thought, if I don't comb it, pull it, or disturb it, the hair won't fall out. As for washing it, I devised an ingenious system. I placed the top part of a stocking on my head and gently pressed the shampoo onto my scalp with my fingertips. Then I stood under the shower for however long it took the last traces of shampoo to fizzle and slide down the drain. And I also did something else. Each time I went for my treatments I tied a very tight band around my head, in an effort to prevent the chemicals from reaching my hairline.

It so happened that I didn't lose a single strand of hair, but this had nothing to do with my silly endeavours. And the other good thing — if I can call it that — about my chemotherapy experience was the lobster dinner that Roy always cooked for me on the days that I had my treatments.

There were twelve sessions of chemotherapy altogether, one treatment every two weeks for six months. And in every instance the scenario was the same. I would be fine for three hours, usually spending this time with my girlfriends, having an extended lunch. Then, as precise as clockwork, I would feel a big crash coming on.

It is quite hard to describe, really. I can tell you what it is *not* — it is not pain. It is more of a disorientation that comes from the conflict between your cognizant and physical self. You feel life ebb from your body, but know that you are not going to die. You feel utterly alone and disconnected from the strangers that you see, who only your eyes recognize as family and friends. Your sense of place, time, and existence becomes murky, but you are fully conscious of everything around you. You desperately search for that one thing that has the power to comfort you.

That one thing — that elixir — I soon realized, was my mother. I wanted to feel her hands, her soft touch caressing my head, my arm, my disfigured chest. I wanted to hear, "There, there, Brenda, everything will be fine. I know. Because I am your mother." And how I cried out for her.

But my mother didn't come. And even in my thirty-eight-year-old mind, I felt that she was abandoning me in my greatest moment of need. Why? Because she had committed the worst act of all. A year earlier she had died.

During this time of wretched debilitation — which would last exactly three days — I merely existed. I kept telling myself that I was doing this for my family, that I had to survive for them. And once I got it into my head that my suffering was in fact a sacrifice for my children, the three days became a lot easier to bear.

Between treatments I tried not to dwell on my illness; I was determined to get back to life as if nothing had changed. But someone in the hospital talked me into joining a support group, and having read that taking part would be a healing experience, I decided to go. There were about ten of us sitting around a table, and everyone, in turn, related their stories. Two of the women even talked about their expected date of demise. Yes, we were all cancer victims, I was thinking, but surely I was not in their league. My heart went out to these women, but I just couldn't handle talk of death at a time when I was trying to focus on recapturing life. After that first meeting I became so depressed that I vowed never to return. I would heal myself my own way.

I thought that keeping busy would work best, and that meant returning to the office, notwithstanding that I was less than halfway through my treatments. I was lucky that my boss encouraged me to come back, willingly accommodating my absences. I rescheduled my eight remaining chemotherapy sessions for Wednesdays so that I could have the weekend to recover from my recurring three-day ordeals.

At work, or anywhere else for that matter, I wouldn't allow my illness to get in the way of the normal course of affairs. I didn't want to be treated differently than before. However, human nature being what it is, I often felt like a circus freak, watching people struggle to move their eyes away from my chest. One man chose to give in to his curiosity, and spent many weeks contemplating which breast was real and which one was the prosthesis. Others, in trying to console me, simply said the wrong thing. I particularly remember one comment from a female colleague. "You know, Brenda," she said, "I could go out there and get hit by a truck." And I said to her, "Me, too. Louise. I could be hit by a truck, too. But I would still have breast cancer."

Slowly, as the novelty of my condition wore off, so too did the curiosity and discomfort of those around me. The "woman with the big C" became Brenda Williamson once again, at least for the next six years. For it was then, in 1995, that I finally went in for breast-reconstruction. And because I took a two-week sick-leave, everyone in the office knew about it.

Reconstruction makes a recurrence harder to detect, and my surgeon had always been dead-set against it. However, I never left my regular check-ups without mentioning it to him. When I passed the five- and six-year marks, my persistence paid off. He reluctantly recommended a plastic surgeon, and the next time he saw me I was reconstructed.

This operation was a watershed in my post-breast-cancer life, and I decided to give myself a treat. I went to a photographer and had a glamour-shot taken, wearing an evening dress with thin spaghetti shoulder-straps and discreetly low cleavage. I hung the photograph in the den, my favourite room in the house, alongside other family pictures. I spend so much time in that room, I wanted it to be a constant reminder of how far I had come since my mastectomy, back in December of 1988.

Upon my return, the women at the office were very excited. No one asked to see my new breast, although I'm sure they wanted to. But, over coffee, polemic on the female body was inevitable. I was quite open about discussing how I felt. I told them that being able to wear a nice bathing suit again would make a big difference in my life. One young woman leaned across the table to within a few inches of me and asked in a hushed voice, as if she were so ashamed on my behalf that she didn't want anyone to hear, "Did you actually go through that operation just to be able to wear a bathing suit?"

"Definitely," I replied. "That's part of who I am. But it is not everything."

I didn't offer any further explanation, although I could tell she wanted to hear more. She was shocked, and looked at me as if I were a traitor to the feminist cause. But I was confident and comfortable with my opinion. I know that having a nice body makes me feel good about myself, and this ultimately determines my quality of life.

My only problem with the reconstruction was the pronounced scarring of the tissue around my breast. The plastic surgeon looked into it, to see if something could be done, but he came up empty-handed. The hard, black ridges, known as keloid, are a common response to cosmetic and other invasive surgeries among most people of African origin. Over the years, however, I've come to view it simply as a scar.

***

As I mentioned before, from the time I was ten years old, living with my brother and three sisters at Aunt Vena's house, I felt a sense of responsibility toward my family, and later it was taken for granted that "Brenda will do it," "Brenda will take care of it," "Brenda will fix it." Why me? Because I've always been able to deal calmly with issues. I've never pounded tables, exploded, or screamed so hard that the veins in my neck swelled up. So when breast cancer came into my life, I tried to approach it the way I had approached all my problems, although, I must admit, emotions were always smouldering beneath the surface.

My first big shock was that I had fallen victim to breast cancer in the first place. People of my ethnicity have heart-related diseases — high blood pressure, strokes, heart attacks. They have diabetes or glaucoma, as I do. Black women do not get breast cancer.

Of course I quickly found out that Black women *do* get breast cancer. They just don't talk about it — not to family, not to friends, not within their community. Breast cancer, much to my regret, remains a very big secret. Body image is so ingrained in our culture that we pass it from generation to generation. When I was growing up, for example, I never saw my mother in anything less than her slip. And, by and large, I continued this behaviour with my own three daughters.

Perhaps this need for privacy comes from the pride that we take in our bodies. So when we get breast cancer, we become ashamed. We keep quiet about it for fear of being ridiculed. In our personal relationships, we think that our men may look at us as failures.

At the beginning I, too, believed that something was wrong with me, that I had been diminished in some way. And I wasn't sure whether I was the one keeping away from Roy, or if he was backing away from me. I knew that Roy was hurting, but I felt completely helpless. A man wants to take charge of a problem, fix it, and forget about it. There is nothing about breast cancer that a man can either fix or forget.

Roy and I never discussed my illness. Only his unusually quiet behaviour at our sessions with the specialists, before my surgery, gave me insight into his real feelings. He was taken aback by the fact that the doctors wanted to remove my entire breast; he, like I, just wanted the lumps taken out. I suppose he was thinking about the aesthetics from his point of view, and he had every right to do so. He wanted to save me from what we both imagined would be certain deformity.

Being ten years older and ten years wiser now, I am much more open about breast cancer than I used to be. This is not to say that breast cancer is the first topic I would raise at a cocktail party, but if the need arises, I do not hesitate to talk about it.

A couple of weeks ago a friend wanted me to talk with a young woman in her twenties who had had a mastectomy a few weeks earlier. She was experiencing a lot of physical pain and emotional anguish. I told my friend I would be happy to help but quickly learned that this would not be easy. My friend wasn't supposed to know about the young woman's mastectomy, and neither was I. In the end I was introduced to her as a friend of her aunt's — a woman I had never met before. I talked to her about my physical experience. About chemo and those three awful days afterward. And I also tried to explain the importance of allowing friends and family into our lives, even if it felt unnatural.

I told her about my eldest daughter, Tafadzwa, who, although not one for many words, always gave me great inner strength. In fact, one day she asked her entire school to pray for me.

In addition, one sister, a flight attendant, was able to visit regularly and kept me distracted with tales of her busy life. Another darling sister, a nurse, who I am convinced missed her true calling as a comic, ran up large telephone bills from Switzerland and kept me laughing. My eldest sister travelled from London to be with me during my chemotherapy sessions and my brother and his wife, who lived close-by, kept tabs on my progress and supplied me with new information on cancer treatments. When a group of friends organized a dinner party shortly after my final chemo session, I felt special. I needed pleasant and positive thoughts to help me beat cancer and ward off bouts of depression. After I had finished talking to the young woman, I am certain that she realized the importance of coming out of hiding.

I feel it is my duty to raise awareness about this disease every chance I get, for as long as there is no cure, our best hope for a long life lies in early detection. Black women must treat breast cancer with the same respect as other killer diseases. Regular check-ups, mammograms, and breast self-examinations should become a routine part of every Black woman's health regime.

Of course I recognize that cultural attitudes are not easy to change. But we all have to become more open. Our lives may very well depend on it.

Afterword

As victims, we all feel the urge to attribute this disease to something in our lives, to fill in the gaps that the medical community has not, to date, been able to. No one can tell us what causes breast cancer — at best, we are given risk-factors that we can rarely do anything about. This means that we must fend for ourselves in trying to escape the groping tentacles of a recurrence.

Once I had ruled out family history, I started to think about my personal life. I had walked my share of rocky roads, to be sure. The divorce back in

1976 wasn't easy, and there were some real tough times with the girls, especially when teenage angst and raging hormones defined all communication between us. I didn't help myself, either, with my constant commitment to other people's problems, small and large. There was the time I rushed to a friend's home with a bag of baby clothes because she had just given birth, and her baby had chronic diarrhea. And there was also the time I went to be with my mother in Jamaica (my parents had moved back there when my mother became ill). Then two months after my mother died I returned again, to arrange for my father's funeral.

I have never been able to get over my parents' deaths. No matter how old you are or how many siblings you have, when your parents die you become an orphan. I grieved for my parents for two years before I was diagnosed with breast cancer. And, even then, the grieving never stopped.

There is nothing I can do about the past. I can, however, try to shape my future. Once, on a visit to Jamaica, I met a very interesting German woman who initially struck me as a relic from the sixties, although she was only forty. She was into watching birds and stars, not television, and her bedroom was plastered with posters that said, "I love myself" and "peace" and "patience." Those were the first things she saw when she woke up. She always said what was on her mind and, in the housing development where she lived, everyone thought of her as "just a weirdo." Maybe she was. But she also exuded great inner strength and an intense level of awareness about her surroundings and herself.

She was a woman of great courage and I wish to become more like her. I think we should all have that aim, to not let society influence us, to put ourselves first for a change, to make up our own rules, to turn off the news. And to develop the art of positive thinking, always taking time out to thank God for His goodness. All these things lead to a long and healthy life.

Gilda Neri

Winnipeg, Manitoba
Date of birth: September 18, 1946
Date of diagnosis: June 1995

To me the worst thing in the world is having breast cancer and not having any money. You can't do anything and you can't buy anything. I'm not talking about going out and things like that. I'm talking about the necessities I can't afford. Going without my vitamins sometimes. That's tough.

I wasn't always poor, and I certainly don't like being poor. I just trusted the wrong person and lost everything.

But I'm doing okay now. I'm going to make it. No matter what has happened to me in the past, I've always been positive about life. And I'm not saying this to show off or anything, but for me breast cancer was just another challenge.

***

When I felt a lump in December 1994, I kept putting off seeing a doctor. I thought it would disappear like the first one had about ten years earlier. I discovered a lump then too, in the same breast, and it went away. Also, since my doctor had moved to a different province, I didn't have a regular G.P., and I didn't feel like seeing a stranger. You know how it is. I didn't want her to think I was whining in case the lump turned out to be nothing. Because when you're poor, you always have to watch how you behave.

The lump was still there in the summer, six months later, so I finally decided that I had waited long enough. I went to the clinic and found out that the doctor who had taken over my G.P.'s practice was a man. This bothered me. Male doctors are just not the same. I mean, granted, they've gone to school and everything, but we're talking about *our* bodies here, and they don't have any experience with that. They're men. They don't have periods. So I asked the receptionist to give me a female doctor.

My new doctor was very nice — in fact, all my doctors are one hundred percent in my book — and she sent me for a mammogram right away. I knew I was in trouble when they had to do it over and over again, six times. I have small breasts, see? And they couldn't get a clear picture. Later, I went to see a surgeon who did a needle biopsy. I saw the blood and that was it.

The whole thing was a shock. I couldn't understand why this was happening to me. I kept on asking, why me? It wasn't that I felt sorry for myself or anything like that, because I was used to having bad things happen. It was that I hadn't done anything wrong in my life. I don't smoke and I don't drink. I've always been good that way. My husband, all my sisters-in-law, and most of my friends smoke and drink. If we have a party at our house, I always have to open the windows afterwards, even if there's a snowstorm outside. See, they do this thing with their cigarettes. They blow smoke-rings out of their mouths, and sometimes they have a contest to see who can blow the most without stopping. Just looking at them makes me choke. So if anyone around me was bound to get cancer, I always figured it would be one of them. Not me.

When I was told about the cancer, the way I looked at it, I only wanted to have the chemotherapy and no operation. But the surgeon was an older gentleman who specialized in breasts, and he explained to me that I didn't have a choice. The lump was large and it had to be scraped out. He thought the best thing for me would be a mastectomy. In the end I was okay with that. I accepted it. And right after the operation, I said to myself, "Hey, I'm in the hospital. I'm strong. I'll make it."

Three weeks after the surgery, I began my chemo. The oncologist said that I could take either the four- or six-month treatment. When I talked it over with my girlfriend, I decided on the shorter one, although I was told it was stronger. But I didn't care. I just wanted to have it over and done with.

Let me tell you, during those four months of chemo, I was a basket-case. Mentally, I was okay, after I decided to shave my head — I thought that one big shock would be better than many smaller ones. But physically, it was very hard, as if some alien had taken over my body, and there was nothing I could do to get rid of it. Nothing to make myself feel better. There were awful sores in my mouth, and I had haemorrhoids. I was sick all the time. And with adriamycin you lose all your hair, everywhere. Eyebrows, eyelashes, armpits, legs, even your private parts. The worst is the head, though, because everyone can see that, even under a wig or a scarf. A bald head is a sure sign of cancer. Once, when we went camping and it was very hot, I couldn't stand to have anything on my head, even though I was surrounded by people. When they saw me, they just walked away with real scared looks on their faces. I didn't say anything. You learn to live with these things.

The hardest part was always the couple of days after each treatment when all I could do was lie in bed and think about my responsibilities, especially what I should be doing for my kids. What made the whole thing rougher on me was that I didn't have any family in Canada. My mother came here once, but decided she didn't like the weather and went home. My mother, my brother, my aunts and uncles are all back in the Phillippines, and my husband's family is just not the same. Oh, they'd come over to visit, but I couldn't rely on them for the really important things, like helping with the shopping and the cooking. Anyway, I didn't want to see anybody. Visitors don't know how to deal with you when you're sick, and you don't know how to deal with them.

If you have support from your family, your friends, your partner, you can handle breast cancer — anybody can — as long as you put your mind to it. But not having relations around, and then on top of that, not having any money, makes it a lot harder. You can ask your own family for financial help, but you can't ask your husband's family or your friends. At least, I can't. Financially, I was on my own. I worried about paying the rent, buying things for my kids, everything. And I was too sick to work. This isn't good. You have to be free of stress, you have to be "happy," in order to cope with your treatments.

I am usually a very positive person, but while I was getting my treatments, I think my husband thought I would croak. Sometimes this got me down, and I even told my kids that if their father found some other woman, I expected them to be nice to her.

Generally, though, Rolly was supportive during my illness, so I can't complain about that. I know some husbands who are not that great. I think men don't understand how sensitive women can get when they've just been told they have breast cancer. If you're healthy and your husband says something you don't like, it's okay, you can take it. When you're sick and he says the same thing, you take it differently, as if it were targeted at you just because you have this disease.

A friend told me about something that her husband did to her, and she is an educated woman. I think her husband has a Ph.D. They were invited to another couple's house for dinner just when Dotty was recovering from surgery. When the hostess brought out coffee and poured everyone a cup, Dotty didn't want any, but she was polite and took a couple of sips. Her husband finished his coffee fast and asked for another cup. Then Dotty said to him, "Take mine, I haven't touched it," and her husband replied, "No thanks. I don't want to drink from your cup." Well! Dotty had a fit. She started to scream that cancer is not catching, and demanded to know how he could behave this way. She said it just came out. She couldn't help it. Her husband got pretty irritated himself, I guess because he thought Dotty was really calling him stupid or something, and he yelled back at her. He said that after twenty years of marriage she should know that he never drinks out of her cup when it has lipstick all over it. He can't stand that. But Dotty spent fifteen minutes in the bathroom crying her heart out. I wonder what the other three talked about when she left them sitting at the table.

My point is that if this can happen to a sophisticated couple, it can happen to anyone. Men have to realize that life is not normal after you've been diagnosed. This is a very sensitive time, and if they really care about their wives, they should watch what they say and how they behave.

Women relate to you differently, whether they've had breast cancer or not. I was lucky to have the support of my best friend, Lina, who never left my side. I remember when I first phoned to tell her the news. I was still talking to her when the doorbell rang, and there she was. I didn't realize that I'd been talking non-stop! By the way, Lina is a Canadian, and she's the one who took me to the doctor and came with me for my chemo.

I also have three other Canadian friends who are great. I can call them in the middle of the night if I want to, and they don't mind. I know I'm lucky because I've met many women who don't have that, who are all alone.

And when you've got little kids to take care of, your situation is really hard. I think my kids had it the worst. They only see things in black and white. Not only was I sick, but my husband was laid off at the time, my unemployment insurance was running out, and we were having some relationship problems. Life is tough enough on kids who come from interracial families without having all these other things happening in their lives.

My kids were only eleven and eight at the time. The older one, my son, told me that he knew how difficult it was for me, but it was very hard on him, too. He wouldn't stop crying. From then on I talked to my kids every night. You know, quality time. I told them that I was fine now, that the cancer was gone, and that even though I was getting sick from the treatments, I would eventually recover. Many times I said that even if something were to happen to me (which wasn't likely, but just in case), I'd make sure they were taken care of. Sure they had their father, but I think they identify with my side of the family more. Besides, my husband wouldn't have been able to look after them. He's a truck driver and spends most of his time on the road. And when he's home, he certainly doesn't want to babysit.

***

I was born in the Philippines, and I guess you could say I had a pretty awful childhood, for reasons I'd rather not talk about. No one listens, anyway. In my experience, no one believes a Filipino.

I wanted to leave home, so in my last year of high school, a few friends and I decided to come to Canada. That was twenty-six years ago. The garment industry was booming in Winnipeg, and I started working in a factory. Later, I went to a nursing home where the pay was better, but I became sick from the smell of the place. When I had a chance at a good, steady job working at a hospital sterilizing surgical equipment, I had to refuse that, too. The smell of the chemicals was the same as in the nursing home. It made me just as sick.

I'm not a shy person and I love people, so I thought I would try bartending and waitressing. I didn't make a lot of money, but I made many new friends. I had a great time. I was single, and I could do anything I wanted. This was certainly more appealing than working in the hospital. Even today, breast cancer and all, I love to party. I think it's very important to have fun in your life, and a lot of people don't get the chance these days. They're either too poor or too rich.

When I met my husband and had my two kids, they became the centre of my life. I decided to return to a part-time job at the garment factory, to be able to get home early in the afternoons to be with them. My husband and I were both working and doing pretty good financially. Of course everything was different then. There were no lay offs and you could always find a job.

In the beginning we had a good life. There was steady cash coming in, and we could go out whenever we wanted. One Christmas we even managed to buy Nintendo for the kids. But I also had my share of challenges. I never had Filipino friends, either because my husband is Canadian or maybe because I don't think the way they do, I'm not sure. And you really can't completely escape from prejudice. I was an immigrant, I had dark skin, I was in an interracial relationship, and I wasn't very educated. I finished high school in the Philippines, but in Canada this is considered equivalent to grade eight or grade nine, at the most.

As the years passed, Rolly spent more and more time at the pub, drinking with his buddies, and this created problems for us. Then our financial situation began to deteriorate with one of us always temporarily out of work. We had a nice little house, but it soon became difficult to both put food on the table and meet the mortgage payments.

In 1992 we hit rock-bottom. We were laid off at the same time and fell three months in arrears at the bank. I approached a friend who had several rental properties in the area (and whose wife was a Filipino, so I thought he could be trusted) and offered him a deal. We would sell him the house for the balance of the mortgage, then rent it back from him as long as he paid our arrears to the bank. He would get a house below market-price, and we would get a break with the rent payments. We didn't want to live for free. We just needed a few months until one of us had work again. This was the deal I thought I signed at his lawyer's office. Well, my so-called friend got title of the house, didn't pay a cent to the bank, and demanded the rent money right away. Meanwhile, the bank was coming after us for the $1,500 in arrears, and in the end, we had no choice. We had to declare bankruptcy.

Rolly didn't blame me for this. Come to think of it, maybe I should have blamed him, because he was drinking too much. But at that point in my life, I only wanted to end the relationship. My problem was that when I told the kids about it, they got very upset. They wanted their father, so I stayed.

I should tell you that my kids always come first with me. Like their schooling. I managed to enroll them in private school, in spite of the fact that we didn't have the money. I was lucky that I found a good Catholic school that was willing to help. They offer partial bursaries for people in low-income brackets, and they let me volunteer, so that I could work off the rest of the tuition fees. I still do this whenever I'm laid off from the factory. I do the lunch programme and field trips, and I even bake perogghis, which is pretty funny for a Filipino, because perogghis are a Ukrainian specialty, really big in Winnipeg because of its large Ukrainian population. So this arrangement with the school works out very well for everyone. The kids are happy there.

I'm lucky that I have good kids. If you have a problem with your kids, public school is better for them. Public schools offer more help, more counselling to those who can't function properly. Some kids have attention deficit disorder, and there is more help available in the public system. In private schools they only concentrate on academic subjects, and all they offer is tutoring.

I am a strong believer in education. Although I realize it doesn't guarantee anything, it increases your chances of having a better life. That's what I tell my kids all the time.

***

When you get breast cancer, finding out you're not the only one really helps. It probably would have hurt a lot more had I thought it was only me.

The best thing that's happened to me since my diagnosis is that I have become involved with a really great organization, called Breast Cancer Action Manitoba. I'm very proud to be a member. There are a few women I don't care for, but that's beside the point. The majority are fantastic. They're the best group. There is a special connection between us and we are all open with each other. You can phone anybody, any time, and it feels like we've known each other for twenty years. Everyone is so compassionate. There are many different types of women, and they all accept you, no matter who you are. I know my standard of living is different from theirs. My husband and I are what some might call "low class." But this doesn't matter. I accept them and they accept me. This is what breast cancer does. It wipes out differences.

In the beginning, when I was having my chemo, it was healing for me to talk with women who had been in the same situation. They helped me to cope and understood what I was going through. And in my case, I had other problems. With the foreclosure and the bankruptcy three years earlier, I was looking for some kind of financial assistance. The group tried to help with that, too, but in the end I couldn't find anything. There was no cancer group or government organization to turn to. And it wasn't as if I didn't want to work. Work is the best thing for everyone. But this situation isn't right. I was sick, I couldn't work, I couldn't take care of myself or my kids. I promised myself then that if I ever won the 6/49 lottery I would buy a rental property and provide housing and amenities for any woman who is poor and has cancer. *I* will become her financial aid, that's for sure.

Now that I'm okay and my breast cancer is in the past, the group is more about socializing with a bunch of women I have something in common with, to get something out of my system if I need to. We joke a lot, we go out for dinners, and there is a lot of information that I get from them which I wouldn't know about otherwise. Some of it is *really* wild. You have to sort it out and find what's right for you. We all have to go with what we believe in.

Sometimes we will have doctors as guest speakers. There was one doctor recently who talked about those other breasts — the reconstructed ones. It was interesting, but I never considered it for myself. It has too many side-effects. I know that having breasts is important for some of the women, but it really doesn't bother me. I'm not a model or anything. When we go camping in the summer, I'm perfectly happy to stay on the grounds and not go to the beach.

Then there is the whole issue of tamoxifen, which we discuss a lot. I found out that tamoxifen sometimes causes blood clots, and increases your chances of getting endometrial cancer. So I told my oncologist that I was really scared because of the varicose veins in my legs. What if I get a blood clot there and they have to cut off my leg? The chance of developing a blood clot is around one percent, my doctor said. Then I asked him, what if that one percent turns out to be me? He said it was a chance I'd have to take. He urged me to consider going on tamoxifen, but I said no. So now I take only vitamins, herbs and nutrients, like Q-10. This is something that a lot of women take in Japan. There was a study done on it, and I know from experience that it really boosts your energy. Whenever I try something new, I always take it by itself for two weeks to see if it works on its own. Then I go back to taking all my other vitamins, herbs, and minerals.

***

Our most important purpose as breast cancer survivors is to do something about this disease. That's our goal. To push as hard as we can to find a cure. And we all do it any way we can.

I saw a video of a speech Dr. Susan Love gave in Montreal, and she said that the only way women can put pressure on the system is by being obnoxious. Because if we irritate the heck out of them, they won't be able to ignore us. They'll do something just to shut us up. I think she's right.

When I joined Breast Cancer Action Manitoba, I didn't like the idea that you meet different members every month. Three, sometimes four or five. They are nice, that's not what I mean, but there are too many of them. Month after month, women in their twenties and in their sixties, black and white, rich and poor, educated and not educated. Now that I've been a member for quite a while, I realize that what's worse than seeing new faces at each meeting is not seeing the regular ones. They are either too sick or they've passed away. To me this says that the medical profession is not doing its job. There isn't enough research. Too many women are getting breast cancer and we still don't have a cure. This disease has been around for a hundred years for all I know, but they haven't found out what causes it. The result is that we all end up diagnosing ourselves, trying to figure out why it happened to us.

Take me, for instance. I'm sure that my own breast cancer was caused by the stress of my financial situation. And since no one can tell me if I'm right or wrong, I have twice the worry. First, I worry about being laid off, and all the financial consequences of that. Then I worry about a recurrence because of getting laid off. I don't want to live like this. I want to enjoy life.

Then there are women who are paranoid. The ones who believe everything in the world is toxic. I don't know, maybe they're right. There's a lot of information on this too, and maybe we are being poisoned by our environment. But until I know for sure, I don't want to live like them either. There's a woman who won't colour her hair — and she's a good-looking woman in her forties — because she is scared of the hair-dye. She won't use nail polish or lipstick or make-up. So she sacrifices the nice things in life because she's terrified.

There are women who spend all their money and time on food. It's one thing to be a vegetarian, but when you get into that expensive organic stuff, and you're too scared to eat even the bread from the bakery or wash your clothes with laundry detergent from the supermarket, there is nothing left of your life. It becomes one hundred percent breast cancer.

Who do I blame for all this? The politicians. There are a lot of big, big politicians who've had breast cancer, yet they've never lifted a finger to do anything about it. Reagan's wife had it when Reagan was president, so why didn't she talk about it? She could have pushed it. What higher person can you ask for than the First Lady of the United States? But Nancy's cause was "just say no" to drugs. I'll never forget those television commercials showing an egg frying in a pan, and the announcer saying, "This is your brain. This is your brain on drugs!" As far as I'm concerned, if we all did our job with our kids so they didn't take drugs, we could put all that money into medical research. The same with Betty Ford. She had breast cancer when her husband was a huge influence in the United States. And what was her cause? The Betty Ford Centre to help rich people who get screwed up by alcohol and drugs. Hey, I know how tough life can be, and I know you can cope with just about anything. And for sure it must be easier when you're rich. So why have all that money wasted instead of putting it to good use? Like finding a cure for those diseases which you don't bring on yourself.

If you ask me, Nancy and Betty and others like them didn't do anything because they were all hypocrites. Had they spoken up twenty years ago maybe something would have been done and we'd know a lot more. Maybe now that Bill Clinton's mom had breast cancer, it will be raised to the right level of awareness.

I don't want to bash one disease for another, but there are many, many more women who get breast cancer than AIDS. And AIDS has only been around since the eighties, not a hundred years. But the progress they've made is ten times greater because the AIDS people are more visible, more powerful than we are, and much louder. They have influential celebrities behind them. We have just ordinary women who must fight very hard, without any funding. Wouldn't it be terrific if we saw breast cancer ribbons instead of AIDS ribbons at the Academy Awards one day? I know someone who's trying to make this happen right now.

It is my prayer that this book will be a best-seller. Then we will have our voice. And, hopefully, everyone will hear us.

Afterword

Whenever someone asks about my life, I ask them how much time they have. Do they want the short version or the long one? The short version is that I was abused as a child, then I came to Canada to make a new life, I lost everything, and I got breast cancer.

The long version is what I have been talking about. But my story is not finished. There are still some things I'd like to say.

On October 7, 1998, it will be three years since I finished my chemo. I am better now and, as far as I'm concerned, I no longer have cancer. So my life is back to normal. At least I want to think it is, but of course it's not. I've lost a breast. And breast cancer is a big part of my life now. So what I really mean to say is that my life is back, but to a different kind of normal, one that will never again be without breast cancer. Sometimes I think about the possibility of a recurrence — but hope and pray it won't happen — and if it does, I'll handle it then. I'm not going to waste my life thinking about it.

Furthermore, I don't ever want to know if I'm dying. I have a friend who was told by her oncologist, right after she finished her chemo, that she would be back in two years time. This isn't a very nice thing to say. The poor woman has given up now. She has no quality of life.

I want to live as if nothing happened, so I'm making plans for my future. I don't have the education to work in an office, but I'm going to make use of my ability to relate to people. I can already see that I'm good at it, because I talk to newly diagnosed women all the time. My doctor gives them my phone number.

What I really want to do is go into business for myself, into sales. There are many entrepreneurs who make a good living. Of course I don't have enough money to start right now, but I will try very hard to make it. I am more determined than I used to be. I want a better life for myself and for my kids. And this time I'll be very careful who I trust.

I should also tell you my husband has really changed since my diagnosis. He still drinks and goes out a lot, because he likes to have fun. And that's okay with me. But he doesn't stay in the pub all day, and he's become a lot more tolerant. Some women I know have bigger problems. They get beat up. At least I don't have that.

If I ever have enough money, I'd like to take a vacation in Mexico with my girlfriend, Lina. We've been thinking about that for a long time. Meanwhile, I'll continue my job at the factory and hope that the economy picks up so that I won't be laid off as much.

But the most important thing is that I'm alive, that I will see my kids grow up, and — I hope — have grandchildren. I may have lost a breast but there are people who have it much worse than me. Those who've lost a leg. Or an arm. Or are in a wheelchair. Maybe I should go to church more often.

Jackie Wasserman

Winnipeg, Manitoba
Date of birth: September 22, 1937
Date of diagnosis: September 30, 1977

In one sense I was lucky. I was spared the anxiety of having to wait for a doctor's appointment. It was my habit to schedule my annual check-up with the gynaecologist around my birthday each year. Other than my children's pediatrician, he was the only doctor I went to see on a regular basis, and this was a good way of remembering to do it. When I got into the bath in preparation for my appointment, I had only one serious concern — how to fake surprise at the breakfast-in-bed ritual that awaited me on the weekend. Maybe my family was planning something special this year. After all, I was hitting the big one. It was 1977, and I was turning forty.

Amid visions of freshly-squeezed orange juice, strawberries and cream, a hot brioche, and a foaming cappuccino, suddenly something awful appeared. Yes, it was definitely there. The lump in my breast was firm and palpable. My heart began to race.

At once the tasks ahead of me took on gargantuan proportions. Getting out of the tub, drying myself, choosing some clothes, putting them on, fixing my hair, applying some lipstick — where's my medicare card? — locking the door. Finally, I was in the car. I turned on the ignition, began to move, and tried to focus my attention on the road. It would be a very long thirty-minute drive downtown.

As soon as I set out I began to sense something familiar. It was what I had felt as a teenager when I had a party to go to Saturday night — and woke up

Tuesday morning to find yet another blemish on my face. I would spend every conscious second of the week obsessing about it, examining the bump from all sides, reassuring myself that it was receding.

But, pimples were long behind me now, and my body was threatening with a much more sinister betrayal. There was a throbbing insistence in my throat, waves of weakness, nausea. I felt the lump from the left, from the right, the bottom, the top, and every other conceivable angle I could manage without crashing the car. Perhaps it was decreasing even as I drove. I thought it was smaller when I touched it from underneath, so maybe that was its actual size. Maybe by the time I arrived at the doctor's it would have vanished altogether.

The gynaecologist immediately sent me for a mammogram and arranged for me to see a surgeon the following week.

I spent that weekend vacillating back and forth, unable to decide whether I had cancer or not. At first I was sure I didn't. Then I changed my mind. The next moment, I had two months to live. Then I convinced myself I was healthy. Yes. No. Life. Death. What will happen to the children? Nothing will happen. Don't worry. You don't have cancer. But, just in case, maybe I should start to make arrangements. All weekend long my mind played snakes-and-ladders with my life. Somewhere in between, I blew out forty candles on a birthday cake.

On Monday afternoon I got the news that there was no carcinoma indicated on the mammogram, but I kept my appointment with the surgeon anyway. I suppose I just didn't like the fact that the lump was still in my body. Thankfully, neither did the surgeon, who insisted on doing a biopsy.

Twenty years ago, a surgical biopsy required an overnight stay in the hospital. The morning after the procedure, I was packing my belongings, making "to do" lists in my head — was Michele's recital on Wednesday or Thursday? — when the surgeon walked into my room with a nurse and a grim look on his face. "I'm very sorry," he began, pausing just long enough to show me the respect most commonly bestowed upon the seriously ill.

The mastectomy would be done as soon as possible, as soon as an operating room became available, he said. In a few days. In the meantime, I would have to remain in the hospital.

There was no way I was going to do that. How could I just stay there, a useless bump on a log? I had to go home. I had to take care of my family. Get

the house in order. Make sure everyone was looked after. Stock the fridge for
their lunch-boxes. Buy groceries. Prepare meals. Write cooking instructions.
Pick up Sigi's shirts from the cleaners.

But in those days, if you were sick, you belonged in the hospital. End of
discussion. So I bombarded my surgeon with the work-in-progress "to do"
list in my head until he gave in. "Let me see what I can do," he replied, and
I smiled in triumph. Then I waited to be told that I could go.

I waited for a day and a half. Finally, word came that they would let me
out for a few hours. But, by then I had spent too much time thinking about
myself. There was nothing in the world, nothing on my mind, nothing in
my soul except breast cancer. My determination had fizzled like the open
cans of soda-pop the kids always left on the kitchen counter. I was
completely self-absorbed, and never made it home.

In the seventies, there was not the same level of awareness of breast
cancer that there is today, or of cancer in general for that matter. Chances
were that you didn't know anyone with cancer, and if you did, it was
someone's great-aunt who had died from it in old age. Statistics were not
public. Causes were not known. It was the affliction of retribution, a
disease of shame. A tragedy. I was in the prime of my life and my kids
were still young. So when all these things conspired against me, I simply
shut down. I stayed and waited for my breast to be cut off. Two days later
it was done.

I had never known loneliness before. As far back as I could remember
I had been surrounded by people. I grew up in a home brimming with
activity, with my parents, my brother, my sister, and a dog named Punch.
It was a busy place, and privacy came at a premium. In my hyperactive
hormone years, I had lots of friends, and we were in constant motion.
Then, after Sigi and I got married, I chose a job that required working with
people. When the children arrived, one, two, three, I found myself at the
centre of the universe.

Now, lying in bed, I felt completely alone for the first time in my life.
Only the sheaf of bandages bore witness to my altered state. I was sedated
for several days.

I had a small group of very good friends with whom I could talk more
intimately, but with most of my visitors, I had to put up a front. I tried to act
no differently than the woman next door who had had her gall-bladder

removed. Our conversations broached safe subjects only — spouses, children, mothers-in-law, the sudden heatwave, the rising star of the Winnipeg Ballet. We talked about everything and everyone under the sun. Everyone, that is, except me. No one dared to ask, and I did not volunteer.

Today, with the benefit of twenty years of hindsight, I know better. I think we all have a visceral need to belong, to be linked in some way to the rest of the world. And when a crisis decimates the landscape of our lives, we need to be recertified by the human race. Ignoring our disease is the same as ignoring us. It is always better to say something, even if it is "the wrong thing," than to say nothing at all.

There was one special person who understood all of this. On the third morning following my surgery, I refused to take any more sedatives. I was awake and alert when I noticed the door to my room slowly open. Someone I had never seen before approached, cautiously taking a few steps. In strong contrast to my own unbalanced disposition, he had a calm and compassionate air about him; I sensed that right away. "How are you feeling, Mrs. Wasserman?" he asked. He was the hospital's chaplain.

At first I replied that I had no need of spiritual guidance. And that if I did, I would call my own rabbi. These were horrible things to say, I know, but the truth is I was angry at the whole world. And that included God. Neverthless, the chaplain sat down at the foot of my bed and, with gentle persuasion, encouraged me to speak. He obviously recognized something I was unaware of — that I needed to talk about my feelings, to vent, to exorcise the pain that clung to the inner wall of my bare chest like a leech.

He was the first person to give me courage, to provide a safe haven in which I could reveal the full extent of my emotions; he was a truly wonderful man. The next day, he came in the morning and again in the afternoon. Soon I'd find myself anxiously pacing the halls waiting for his visits. When the result of my bone scan didn't arrive on time and I was beside myself, he brought it to me. He always listened without judgement. He comforted me. And through our conversations, he gave me the opportunity to begin to heal. I guess I'm still healing because I haven't shut my mouth about breast cancer ever since.

After the surgery, I required no further treatments. The oncologist did not recommend chemotherapy, and radiation was unnecessary because I'd had a radical mastectomy.

Once I got home, I made up my mind to resume a normal life as quickly as my physical recovery would allow. I tried to convince myself that the crisis was over. It was time to move on. But this didn't mean I'd pretend that I'd had a gall-bladder removed instead of a breast. And I wasn't about to go into hiding. I knew that I must talk about it, that for me talking was therapeutic — the chaplain had taught me that. The issue was how to do it right for everyone involved. I had lived my entire life by rote, and now there was no script.

One of my first undertakings was to call the school's principal and let him know what was happening in our lives. I wanted to warn him, should any of the children suddenly develop problems. Actually, this was relatively easy for me to do. From the beginning I had no problem saying breast cancer, and I've often wondered whether, in those days, people cringed more at the word breast than at the word cancer.

My pre-eminent concern was protecting the kids , who were nine, thirteen, and fifteen at the time. And I cursed Dr. Spock. He had advice on every child-rearing issue anyone could think of except how to tell your children their mother has cancer.

When I sat down with my eldest, Jeffrey, he told me that he had just finished a project on Happy Rockefeller for his biology class. Mrs. Rockefeller was the first public person to openly talk about her disease. We had a long conversation then, the first of many to follow, about Happy Rockefeller, and breast cancer, and me. But Jeffrey would not show me that report. He only told me later that he cried when he re-read it. And that broke my heart, because mothers are supposed to make things better, not worse.

My younger son, Trevor, was a very introspective child. He was unable to talk about his feelings even when I tried to coax them out of him. He kept everything inside, and I had to constantly remind myself that forcing the issue only satisfied my needs, not his. Reluctantly, I acknowledged that his way of coping was equally valid, though different, from his brother's.

With my nine-year-old, my daughter Michele, I decided to follow the pediatrician's advice and not tell her anything. In retrospect, this was a huge mistake. It did more harm than all the cumulative mistakes I had made with her to that point in her life. Michele was very conscious of the fact that something was wrong with me. She knew that I'd had some surgery. Everyone around her was whispering, and she was excluded. She changed in front of my eyes from an outgoing, independent child to a withdrawn introvert, who became very clingy and never left my side.

Then there was Sigi. He had a very hard time accepting my illness. When I was still in the hospital and his buddies tried to take him out for a cup of coffee, to let him spill his guts, he turned them down. So I never cried in front of him. I didn't tell him how afraid I was, that there were times when I thought I was going to die. My conscience wouldn't allow me. Nor was I capable of helping him.

My sister's visit from Vancouver, however, was a most refreshing change of pace. I will never forget what she said to me when I picked her up at the airport. After our first hug, she raised her arms to the heavens and exclaimed loud enough for everyone to hear, "Thank God you don't stink of cigarette smoke any more." (I quit the day I was diagnosed.) A few minutes later, when we were driving home, she said something about how amazing it was to see me coping so well.

I told my sister that I don't think any of us knows what we will or won't do, or how we will or won't react to a particular situation in our lives. Me give up? Never. I had come close just once, that time in the hospital, before my mastectomy, when they wouldn't let me go home.

"You're doing just fine without me," my sister said one day as she cut her visit short. After she left I returned to work part-time. I hadn't completely recovered from the surgery, but work was my bridge back to the real world; from then on, life seemed to proceed in an orderly fashion, more or less.

***

I don't mean to leave you with the impression that I got over this egregious event in my life in just a few weeks. I didn't. But what I remember most is how hard I tried. In fact the aftermath of breast cancer, it seems to me, has a unique life of its own. It gets its second wind after the doctors are through with you. It infiltrates your mind and, I'm sad to say, doesn't ever leave completely.

In the beginning we eat, drink, and sleep the fear of a recurrence, and I was no exception. Then, one day, a moment comes when everything looks bright and positive, and we can stop holding our breath. With time, these moments of confidence become longer and longer, and it is the fear that becomes a fleeting, idle thought.

Many women draw on an entirely new set of assumptions about life, about themselves and their relationships, in order to put themselves on fast-forward. For me, getting back to the routine of daily life worked best. I was intent on keeping busy, more than ever, in order to prevent a free thought from entering my head.

Two and a half years after my mastectomy, in 1980, after I thought I was way past the fear, I developed very bad pains in my arms. I knew it wasn't lymph edema, so it had to be metastases — what else! I ran to the oncologist. He was unable to find anything specific, but when we sat in his office face-to-face, and I was quiet and calm once again, he looked at me with avuncular concern and said, "If you were my wife, Jackie, I would insist on having your other breast removed." He based his opinion on the density of my breast and the fact that my particular cancer, should it recur, would not respond to chemotherapy. The alternative was to live the rest of my life under constant medical surveillance — monthly examinations, blood-works, ultrasounds — waiting to catch the cancer in time. And even that was not a full guarantee.

It took me six months to make up my mind.

Without a doubt, this period of procrastination was the most difficult of my life. It wasn't anything like the panic or the self-pity I had felt the first time. Rather, I just couldn't accept the brutality of my options. Either way I would lose. Lose another breast to save my life, or lose the life I had known, lived, and loved to save my breast.

I knew this needed to be *my* decision, but I was desperate for someone to help me make it. I had to find a reason, anything, for going one way or the other. I went from doctor to doctor, four altogether, but became none the wiser. I contacted the cancer society. I talked with girlfriends, who, in truth, qualified only because they had breasts.

Maybe all I needed was for someone to tell me, "Jackie, you are a wonderful person, and we love you, whether you have two breasts, one breast, or none." Maybe I should have asked louder for help, for it seemed no one around me was listening.

Nor did I want to involve my husband, Sigi. I never wanted to be in a position to blame him should I eventually become unhappy with whatever choice I had made.

Finally, a friend who was a nurse helped me put things into perspective. The logic had always been there, but I hadn't been able to find it amidst the commotion. It seems so simple now. I could live without another breast, she said, but I might not live if I got breast cancer again.

Day and night I thought about that conversation, and although I knew Mary was right, I couldn't find the strength to act on it. I was healthy. I *felt* healthy. The whole situation was so unfair.

It didn't matter who was buzzing about, watching television, talking on the phone, fighting for the shower, giving me their laundry, calling me "mom," or "sweetheart," or "Jackie-oh," or blasting me for my luck in a game of monopoly. I was alone. I knew that I could rely on no one but myself.

I gathered all my inner resources and went to see a plastic surgeon. There were several possibilities, I was told, the most promising of which was a new technology that had been remarkably successful in healthy women seeking breast enhancements. Shortly after my meeting with this man, I made up my mind. But my decision to go ahead with the second mastectomy was very much tied to having reconstructive surgery.

Just before I entered the hospital, I decided to sit down with my daughter, Michele, and explain to her what was going on. The time was right. By then she was almost twelve, racing rapidly towards puberty. I focused on issues of feminine identity, which took the pressure off the more serious matter — the one about breast cancer being a potentially fatal disease.

I went for the surgery in June of 1980, and it turned out that the oncologist had been right. My other breast was pre-cancerous. I had been sitting on a time bomb. Who knows if the cancer would have been caught in time? Thank God I had an oncologist who cared. I owe him my life.

Five months later I underwent plastic surgery. I was the plastic surgeon's first patient for bilateral, Dow Chemical silicone breast-implants.

I've always had very large breasts. "Well-endowed," they used to say when I was growing up. But after the implants, my breasts were so small that I had trouble finding a well-fitting bra. Exasperated after yet another unsuccessful trip to the lingerie department, this time to Eaton's, Michele came to my rescue. "Hey mom, do you want to borrow my training-bra?" she asked, marking our entry into the next level of the mother-daughter relationship — clothes swapping. I knew then that Michele was out of harm's way.

Knock on wood, in the eighteen years that have passed, I've had no problems, either on the cancer front or with the silicone breast-implants.

***

Looking back now, I realize just how different my life has become as a result of my experience. During my first forty years, I was a traditional, middle-class wife. I married at twenty, got a job, raised three kids, cooked, baked, and socialized. We went to the movies on Saturday nights, and I played *mahjong* with a group of women once a week. The universe was unfolding according to plan. Then everything changed.

After breast cancer, many things were suddenly no longer important. Like keeping an impeccably clean house. Or doing things because they were expected of me. I recognized that I, too, had needs and the right to fulfill these needs, although it wasn't immediately clear to me what these needs were. My role as the family's primary caregiver was fundamental. I accepted that. I am not a Jewish mother for nothing! But this was not my life's only purpose.

In 1981 I was asked to participate in a pilot project for the Cansurmount programme of the cancer society, and I realized that there was a whole other world out there with lots of wonderful people in it. We shared many common bonds. I discovered how gratifying it was to be part of a network that provided desperately needed, emotional support to others, and I've been a volunteer with them ever since. The opportunities I've had and the help I've been able to offer are gifts I can't possibly measure. I have learned that whatever you give of yourself, whatever you do for others, comes back to you a million times over.

However, being an advocate for cancer support will be important only as long as it remains important to me. Something else may come along, and if I find it appealing, I will take that on too. Part of growing as a human being, I believe, is the ability to discern, to become comfortable with yourself, to recognize that being an "I" centred person is a moral obligation, not a vice.

Unfortunately, many would be quick to disagree. I recently met someone who, until breast cancer, had been a successful corporate executive. She is an artist now. We talked late into the night, enjoying the kinship that comes from a shared, deeply personal experience. Two amateur philosophers solving all the ills of the world — the world according to breast cancer.

At one point, she related a recent conversation with her husband of fifteen years. He isn't at all pleased that she has changed careers mid-stream. He told her that he feels betrayed, that when he married her, it was on the assumption they would pursue a common dream. He was smitten with a promising corporate star, not a starving artist, and she is breaking their implicit marriage contract. In her defence, my newfound friend told her husband that breast cancer was not included in their marriage contract either. He should be proud of the fact that she has grown. Her husband replied, "You haven't grown. You've just changed."

He is wrong. Personal growth is all about looking into yourself, spreading your wings, taking risks, trying something new, exploring what you, as a human being, have, are capable of, and need.

Regretfully, I'm aware of many similar stories, and some that are worse. One woman's husband told her that she was so ugly now he never wanted to look at her again. And I did an open-line radio show once about breast cancer survivors whose husbands had left them. There were so many women that we couldn't handle all the calls. It was terrible.

Here is my amateur version of why this happens: as breast cancer survivors, most of us know that we have been irrevocably changed by our disease. We look through different glasses, we think different thoughts, we choose different friends, we feel what others cannot. We are on a journey toward self-knowledge. The unfortunate part is that many of our partners don't make this journey with us. They haven't had our experience. Or, they choose not to make it. In either case, it is not our responsibility to teach them. It is their responsibility to learn.

Eventually, if one person grows and the other doesn't, the disparity becomes too great, and the one who stayed behind runs away. Probably as much from himself as from his wife.

Afterword

Breast cancer is an experience of contrasts. It is enemy and friend, an end and a beginning, sorrow and joy. This is how it leads us on the journey toward self-knowledge.

We each embark on this journey at a time that is right for us. In my case, it took almost four years from when I was initially diagnosed. For my artist friend, however, it took less than a few hours.

Common to all travellers is that we never reach our destination. We only encounter signposts along the way. I consider myself extremely lucky that rather early on I came across one that read: "what feels right, *is* right. Follow your heart. Explore every avenue that is important for you." This credo guides all aspects of my life, everything I do. It has brought me immeasurable happiness and is the most valuable insight that I can pass on.

Delores Bartel

Calgary, Alberta
Date of birth: September 15, 1944
Date of diagnosis: June 29, 1993

This story is not only about breast cancer; it is about my life. I must therefore begin with the most influential figures: God, with whom I have a fifty-four year relationship; my husband, who has been by my side for forty years; and of late, my plastic surgeon, who put me back together after cancer took both my breasts.

All my life I had been noticed for my breasts, they were a big part of my identity. By the seventh grade — when Lana Turner and Jayne Mansfield were the icons of the times — I was already a C-cup, and had been branded the girl that other girls envied. To kids my age, I was different. It didn't matter a hoot that I came from a strict Mennonite home and went to church every Sunday; my reputation was compromised by my bra-size.

I always dreaded gym class, anticipating the worst from my classmates, and one of the turning points of my early years came in the aftermath of yet another insensitive prank. I can still see myself sitting on the bench in the locker room, resolved to come to terms with my genetic makeup. It occurred to me that I had two choices in life. I could bend over, hump my back and dissolve into anonymity, or I could lose my inhibitions and accept my body with pride. I walked out of school that day holding my head high, too young to recognize that my real commitment was to resilience in the face of adversity.

Forty years down the road this resolve would prove invaluable in my battle with breast cancer, the most formidable adversary I have ever had to face.

***

The first person I knew who got breast cancer was Norma, and my story really begins with her.

Norma and I had known each other since we were kids, growing up in the same small town in rural southern Alberta. We were both in our late thirties when Norma was diagnosed, back in 1982, and I couldn't understand it. Her breasts were like two raisins on a breadboard. How could she have breast cancer with those things?

Her diagnosis came as a shock to everyone. I saw her many times, especially when she was in the hospital, but it was difficult for us to be intimate. We didn't have that type of relationship, and I raised the issue of her illness only when I sensed she wanted me to. At one point I mustered up my courage to ask her why she had gone for a breast exam in the first place — in those days breast exams were the exception, not the rule. When Norma said that she had known in her heart something was wrong, I knew what she meant. I worried about my breasts all the time; they were so lumpy, bumpy, and big — with plenty of room for cancer to take hold.

Norma's illness hit me deep. But, to be honest, I was also very concerned for myself. What if this were to happen to me? It would be the most horrible thing in the world.

Then Norma died, and I felt guilty, because my personal fears somehow seemed to diminish my sorrow for her tragedy. I later realized, of course, that this wasn't the case. When I cried, it was for Norma, for me, for all of us.

I always think about Norma with gratitude. Because of her, I began to listen to my body, to become familiar with every membrane in my breasts. I had mammograms yearly, sometimes six months apart, whenever my instincts told me to. My all-too-frequent check-ups usually included a breast exam. I learned to recognize when something didn't feel right, and I acted on it. If breast cancer was to be my destiny, I had to do everything in my power to catch it in time.

The first suspicious lump showed up when I was about forty, and it required a surgical biopsy. It was a scary, almost mystical experience, shrouded in secrecy, because the surgeon didn't explain anything beforehand. I had no idea what to expect, so before I was put under, I tried to deflect the gravity of the situation with a little humour, saying "Please remember to leave some darts and tucks in case I need to have them filled up again." But the surgeon didn't laugh. In fact, he didn't react at all. I suspect he felt insulted.

However, over the next few years, Dr. Y. and I became comfortably acquainted, and on the occasion of my second biopsy, it was he who raised my couturier concerns. "Still the same request about the stitching, Delores?" he asked, smiling behind his surgical mask. "You bet," I replied.

Once again, the biopsy was negative.

This constant medical attention — including incidents that required hospitalization — did not merely mitigate my worries; it liberated me from them. This was the only way I could live. And except for the occasional panic attack, my life was like something straight out of a Harlequin romance, with a cast of characters that included Sieg, two beautiful children, and "Grandpa."

***

I was fifteen when I met my husband, Siegfried, on a province-wide youth retreat organized by churches across Alberta. 1960 was a leap year, which meant that the girls got to choose their guys for the Saturday-night social. I picked Sieg, of course. He was not much of a looker, and at twenty-two, the age difference between us was huge, but the moment I laid eyes on him, I knew he was the man I'd marry. According to him, when he first saw me in my mother's sweater, he knew he was in trouble. Our wedding took place a year and a half later, the day after my seventeenth birthday.

Sieg had come to Canada from East Germany, and held firmly to his European upbringing. He believed that if he couldn't take care of a wife, he didn't deserve to have one, and so I became barefoot and pregnant, raising our two daughters, who were both born before I turned twenty-one. Being a mother was my most important role.

Business success came early for my husband, and soon we were able to join those fortunate enough to flee the Canadian winter. On our first trip to Maui, we befriended an old Hawaiian who did odd jobs around the hotel. "Grandpa," as we came to call him, was poor and newly retired, and his family appeared to have little use for him. But he was a very gentle man and became our host. He took us around the islands to places ordinary tourists never see, allowing us to experience Hawaii through his native eyes.

We were returning to Calgary for the Christmas holidays and we invited Grandpa to come with us. He had never left home before, and the idea of a white Christmas in the middle of the Canadian Rockies captivated him. But he would only come if he could pay for his own airfare. Sieg and I were relaxing on the beach, sipping our pina coladas, when we saw Grandpa running in the distance, waving the plane ticket in his hands, yelling "Baby, baby," (his term of endearment for me) "I'm going to see the snow!" It was a close call. We were leaving the next day.

Calgary didn't let us down that year. The city was enshrined in white, and Grandpa was bewitched, by the snow, the fur coats, the rubber galoshes — too heavy to fish in, he said — the touques, the mittens, and the rest of our winter paraphernalia. His favourite pastimes were sledding with the girls and listening to Bing Crosby Christmas LPs. He wanted to learn to ski. What can I say? We adopted him.

For close to twenty years, we spent six months of the year in Calgary and six months in Maui, where Grandpa occasionally would see his other family. I lived in the happily-ever-after of a fairy tale. I ran two households and raised our daughters according to solid, old-fashioned, European values, which — by no coincidence — I shared with Sieg. I had my Mom, Dad, and Grandpa to take care of, my in-laws to nurture, and social functions to host. We loved each other so much that Sieg and I often spent twenty-four hours a day together.

Threaded throughout these years were the visits with my doctors. When I got the all-clear from them, my life became perfect again.

***

In 1988 my first grandchild — a little girl — was born. The first time I held her in my arms I was flooded with images of my own grandmother, and the only thing I could remember about her was her size. That I had been fat was not something I wanted Amanda to remember about me, and her birth inspired me to finally do something about it.

I joined Weight Watchers, and after I had reached my goal weight, I was asked if I'd be interested in becoming a meeting leader. Since I hadn't worked outside the home before, I thought a part-time job would be nice. I was forty-four years old, not even a high school graduate (I married Sieg after the tenth grade), and this seemed a wonderful opportunity. Furthermore, I had the time. Grandpa had passed away, the girls were living their own lives, both married now, and when Amanda was born, I had decided I would never become a grandmother who did nothing but babysit.

My first time in front of an audience, I faltered, but only for a moment. Then I felt a sudden rush of energy. It came from the power of my convictions, just like that day so many years before in the locker room. It was an exhilarating feeling. Everyone was listening to me! Using my personal experience to help others appealed to me, satisfied my heart and soul. With my job, I was complete.

***

Five years later, in 1993, a third breast-incident snuck into my life. I had a good track record behind me and felt confident after the procedure, this time a needle aspiration.

Then came the phone call. I was home briefly between Weight Watchers meetings, and I can still see where I was sitting, what I was reading, what I was wearing the moment I heard Dr. Y. say, "Delores, I have some bad news for you." I took a breath, and it stuck in my throat. For an instant, I didn't know how to exhale. In just a few seconds, dozens of thoughts ran through my mind. My biopsies are always negative. They must have made a mistake. No, they didn't. I'm going to die. How will I tell my husband? I want to see my grandchildren grow up. What if I've passed this terrible disease on to my daughters? I'm going to get through this. But Norma didn't. Because hers was caught too late. What if mine has been caught too late? We're supposed to be eating out with friends tonight. Will I lose my breast?

With this *Laterna Magica* show reeling in my head, the only words I could manage were, "Now what?" It was a visceral, rather than gracious response to my long-time surgeon.

After he explained the process and I had hung up the phone, I just sat there, alone, and for the longest while, time stood still. I went to my afternoon meeting, but I don't remember how I made it there, what I said, or how I drove home. At that point I hadn't told a soul. I delayed calling my daughters, waiting instead for Sieg to come home. I wanted him to be the first to know.

Dr. Y. removed a mass the size of a goose egg, which left only a hollow in my bra that was easy enough to fill with a little padding. I was comfortable with that. I didn't feel disfigured, and I certainly didn't feel any less of a woman for it. Sieg loved me just the same. He used to say that he cherished that breast the most, "my poor little boob," because it had gone through so much.

The cancer was *in situ*, and I was put on tamoxifen. No chemotherapy, no radiation. That sounded great in the beginning, but within a few months I found myself putting on weight and becoming more and more worried about it. When I discussed this with the oncologist he couldn't supply a satisfactory explanation. Perhaps women become distraught over their diagnosis and overeat to compensate, he said. However, the doctor was adamant that there was no medical connection. I was very apprehensive listening to this, but I chose to believe him. If my weight gain was caused by tamoxifen, there was nothing I could do about it. On the other hand, if it was emotionally induced — and, incredibly, I wasn't aware of my own behaviour — I certainly had all the tools at my disposal to deal with it. For goodness sake, I'd been teaching this stuff for years.

To my utter dismay, none of my tools worked. Furthermore, I loved my job, but in order to keep it I couldn't go above my goal weight, and I didn't have a clue what to do. Other than my oncologist, there was no one I could ask for help. I was supposed to be the help. Then it occurred to me that there must be hundreds, thousands, even tens-of-thousands of women in the world in my situation. Perhaps they come to our meetings frustrated that they're doing everything right but just can't lose the weight. And all because of tamoxifen! One way or another, I was going to find a solution. I would save the world.

One year later, my mission was sidetracked when I discovered a lump in my other breast. I would wake up in the mornings and find my hand cupping it. In bed, at night, the last thing I would do was check if the lump was still there. When this activity turned into an obsession (which didn't take too long), I called Dr. Y.

Dr. Y. examined me the following morning and scheduled yet another biopsy, this time to be done under a local anaesthesia. I hated the idea of being cut open, while wide awake and alert. It reminded me of going to the dentist. I'd be able to hear and see everything, and I wouldn't escape the pain; it would all be right there, inside my head. Before the procedure, I asked my doctor for a sedative — not that it helped.

Dr. Y. removed the lump, no larger than a thumbnail, and showed it to me. It looked good, he said, but he continued to cut. I can still hear that awful crunching noise as he snipped at my breast, piece after piece, asking his assistant for more vials, his calm demeanour progressively unravelling, telling his assistant to rush the samples directly to pathology.

Afterwards, I was sent to the recovery room to wait for the sedative to wear off. I was waiting, not too patiently, when a nurse approached holding a syringe in her hand. She asked if I wanted something for the pain. I didn't understand. I had no pain. But I decided to take the shot anyway. I think I already knew. Then Dr. Y. walked in, looking like someone on his way to confession.

Thinking he had come to take me home, Sieg arrived within minutes of Dr. Y. The truth is, I was glad he heard it from the doctor. It had been difficult for me to tell him the first time, and I didn't think I had it in me to do it again. My husband's timing was not a coincidence; I knew that. Nothing in life is.

Dr. Y. pulled up a chair beside my bed, as if to avoid looking down at me. Sieg was on my other side. We were holding hands.

It was a serious situation. Another primary cancer, and this time it was ductal. Although he didn't have all the test results, Dr. Y. was certain I would need a double mastectomy.

Sieg tightened his grip on my hand.

"A double mastectomy," I said, "you mean like — gone?"

Dr. Y. nodded. Strangely, my mind wasn't whirling like the last time. At that moment, my only concern was for Sieg. I wanted to tell him I was sorry.

Dr. Y. went on to tell us about a plastic surgeon who had returned recently to Calgary after training in Texas. He had an excellent reputation and used the latest reconstruction techniques. "You may want to think about something like that," he said.

"What's his name?" I asked, as fast as I could get my lips to move.

More out of instinct than a need for approval, I turned my head away from the surgeon to look at my husband. Sieg had been silent until now, trying to absorb what the doctor was telling us. Now it was time for him to speak. And he was calm and deliberate, his voice resonating with all the love I had grown accustomed to in our thirty years together. "Whatever you decide, hon, I'm with you all the way," he said. Whereupon Dr. Y. volunteered to make the appointment.

By ten the next morning, Dr. Y. was on the phone, anxious to tell me about his success. He sounded almost happy. "Delores! The plastic surgeon is willing to squeeze you in during his lunch-hour today."

Without thinking, I told him I couldn't make it. I had a Weight Watchers meeting at noon, and I didn't think I'd be able to find someone to replace me on such short notice.

Silence at the other end. Then, testily, "It's the only time he has," meaning "perhaps you should re-think your priorities."

"I'll be there," I replied.

***

On my way to see Dr. B., I envisaged arriving at a Hollywood movie set, complete with Beverly Hills-type characters. A spacious office in a modern high-rise, with plush carpeting, original paintings on the walls, art deco furnishings, and perhaps a receptionist with a big smile and double-duty mascara. A tall, dark, handsome doctor, greying at the temples, wearing an Armani suit under his open white lab-coat — just three buttons open — a Rolex glowing on his wrist. Everything the way I'd seen on television.

I arrived at a shopping mall and found his office down a side corridor on the second floor. Entering the claustrophobic waiting area, I was greeted by a harried receptionist. She ushered me into a room that looked like a laboratory straight out of a forties B-grade movie. There were strange tools and instruments everywhere, a couple of sinks, used hospital cabinets, and a big, green dental chair with torn cushions. It looked like something bought at a yard-sale. "Oh, Lord," I thought, "this is *not* where I want to be."

When Doogie Howser entered, I was so underwhelmed I couldn't restrain myself from being flippant. Poor Dr. B. He didn't react to my snide remarks, but he certainly blushed a great deal.

The young doctor told me to take everything off from the waist up and to lie down in the chair. (*That* chair?) A few minutes later, he asked me to pull down my pants (all the way to you-know-where), so he could examine how much stomach tissue I had. There I was, reclined half-way in a dental chair, naked except for my non-consequential parts, thinking that this scenario was getting worse by the minute.

Dr. B. was prodding and probing my stomach when he suddenly stopped to stare at my appendectomy scar. I could see concern on his face. "What happened here?" he asked. "It looks like an army surgeon did it." I, of course, had always assumed appendectomy scars were *supposed* to look like mine.

Instant flashback to the appendix attack. "I was fourteen," I said, remembering how terribly upset I had been because I was having my period at the time and the nurses had to change my pads — to a fourteen-year-old girl, perhaps the most embarrassing thing in the world. Then, in my mind's eye, I saw the only family doctor I had ever known: a man from small-town southern Alberta, probably ex-army, who had shown such reckless disregard for the body of a teenager. How could he have done this to me? Sensing my despair, Dr. B. added quickly, "Never mind. I'm sure we can work around it." I breathed easier after that.

"How many people die during breast reconstruction?" I asked, serious this time, as I was putting on my clothes. Dr. B. was non-plussed. "I haven't lost anyone yet," he replied. I left his office and agreed to come back for another consultation. A real appointment this time.

With Dr. B.'s encouragement, I set about doing my homework. I talked with other women about their reconstruction experiences to find out the good, the bad, and the ugly. I went to the library at the Tom Baker cancer clinic and spent my free time reading, learning, and generally becoming knowledgable in the specifics of my case. When I had evaluated all my options and talked them over with Sieg, I felt confident. This was how I wanted it. As for matters relating to Dr. B., everything I heard about him was positive. There was only praise. "Time to drop the flippancy, Delores. Lighten up," I said to myself.

I was in a much better state when I went back for my second meeting. During the time we spent together, I realized that Dr. B.'s main concern was my well-being. He was different from my other doctors. He seemed to care about me on a personal level, and I left his office content with the rapport between us. (But this didn't mean that I wouldn't try to make him blush.)

On my way out, the receptionist stopped me. "Mrs. Bartel. There's something you should know," she said. And as I heard these words, my heart began to pound. When you're dealing with cancer, this usually signals bad news. But then she leaned across her desk and whispered, "The doctor's breasts are masterpieces. Better than the originals."

At home, Sieg and I sat down with our after-dinner drinks and discussed the issue of timing. I could have had my breasts lopped off in an instant, but if I wanted it done the way Dr. B. had presented it to me, I had to wait until an operating room became available. The two combined surgeries would take

anywhere between ten to fifteen hours and would require four physicians —
Dr. Y., Dr. B., his assistant and the anaesthesiologist — plus nursing staff.
The wait could take several months. It was now September.

I think even Sieg was surprised by my attitude. I wasn't in a panic, like the
first time, in spite of the "serious diagnosis." I didn't feel pressured. In the
year since my lumpectomy, I had learned a lot about myself, about the nature
of healing, about breast cancer. I had learned, for example, that you are not
going to die if you don't jump the moment you are diagnosed. You are better
off researching your own case than relying exclusively on what the doctors
tell you. I had a copy of every single lab report contained in my medical files,
and this is not an exaggeration. And I asked questions all the time, no matter
how stupid they appeared to be — like asking Dr. B. how many patients die
from breast reconstruction.

Then, too, I had something else to consider. Before any of this happened,
we were planning to spend the month of November in Maui. Maui had always
been a special place for us. For twenty years, it had served as our second
home. We belonged to a community there; we had friends. Our eldest
daughter got married there. We met Grandpa there. And, I thought, who
knows how long the cancer has been inside my body. If the Lord has kept me
alive this long, an extra month's delay isn't going to do any harm.

When we left for Maui, I had a Prozac prescription with me, but after a
week I stopped taking it. I felt God could do a better job of preparing me
emotionally. I was used to talking with the Lord. That November, in Maui, I
simply talked to Him more often. It was not important for me to understand
why this was happening to me. The real question was where I would go from
here.

Searching for answers, I became more in tune with myself and the world
around me. The sky was a brighter shade of blue, the ocean more mysterious,
the earth's scents and flavours more intense — as was my love for Sieg. I was
in complete harmony with the universe.

***

December 12, 1994: the eve of my surgery. It used to be that you checked
into the hospital the night before an operation. With the cutbacks to the
health-care system, it's not like that any more and it's just as well. This gave
me the opportunity to spend time with myself in the comfort of my own

home. I took a shower, had a good long look in the mirror, and made my farewells, realizing that I would never see, or feel, or touch my breasts again. I had to burn an image of what I looked like into my mind. It was a very private and difficult time, like parting from precious friends. And Sieg was very affectionate that night. I could sense his concern as he caressed me, almost unconsciously. When you've been married as long as we have, that's very special, believe me, because any caressing that goes on after thirty years is always one hundred percent conscious.

December 13, 1994: we arrived at the hospital at six a.m. Dr. Y. came in to say hello. Then Dr. B. took me into a side room. I had to strip naked and stand in front of him while he marked up my body with a black felt-tipped pen. This was when the indignities of illness registered fully in my mind. All those times we "take everything off from the waist up" for breast exams, or "from the waist down" for those unpleasant ultrasounds. Standing stark-naked without being able to pull in my stomach, however, was definitely my lowest point.

When Dr. B. was finished, I felt like a road-map with sweeping strokes of semi-circles, half figure-eights, and ovals all over my body. "We're ready," he said. "It's time to go." Sieg was on my left, Dr. B. on my right, as we headed for the operating theatre on foot. We took the elevator to the second floor and walked down the hall past the pacing room (where patients' relatives wait during surgery). It felt very bizarre. I was used to being rolled into the O.R. on a bed.

Outside the doors of the theatre, I kissed Sieg good-bye. I had spent three months preparing for this moment, and I was going in peace. Sieg, on the other hand, was very pale. He didn't say anything, perhaps because he couldn't. I went through the doors feeling the despondency of his gaze at my back. For the first time in my life, there was nothing I could do for him.

Before I realized it wouldn't be possible, I had planned to leave a little post-it-note for Dr. B. on my tummy. It read, "Dear Dr. B. If you're going to have lunch, please don't leave any crumbs." The post-it was in the trash, but the words were in my head. They were the last to leave my mouth.

Coming out of the anaesthesia, with the flurry and bustle of the recovery room confirming that I was still alive, I immediately focused on my chest. It was more a reflex than a deliberate act. Although I had no bandages, I wasn't able to see very much. My gown was drawn closed and clipped to a machine somewhere behind me that made scary, beeping sounds, and I was too afraid to move. But the rise and fall of two silhouettes was a very good sign. Something was there. I thanked the Lord and closed my eyes. The next time I opened them, I saw my husband's face. The most handsome face I have ever seen.

Dr. B. took six inches from my tummy — which I'm told is a lot — because he wanted to provide me with the exact same D-cup I had been before. When I saw myself in the mirror I couldn't believe it. I had breasts! And today, after nipple reconstruction and tattooing, my breasts look ten years younger. They are beautiful. They don't sag or droop. And there's hardly a visible scar. Whether I am dressed or naked, no one ever knows the difference.

I stayed in the hospital for eight days, and Dr. B. came to see me once each morning and again before he left at night. He was my chaplain, my therapist, and my knight-errant. Not to mention my Master Breast Cancer Magician.

***

The oncologist explained that I had two options for chemotherapy, and I decided on the six-month treatment because I didn't want to lose my hair. I had had enough body alterations. I wanted my life back to normal. What I didn't count on were the differences between what I and others would consider normal.

For me, normal included Sunday dinner after church with our daughters and their families. We've been going to church all our lives, and when the girls got married, Sunday dinner continued to be a family tradition. By 1994 there were ten of us at the table.

One Sunday I overheard my daughters talking between themselves in the kitchen within earshot of Amanda. During dinner Amanda thrust her seven-year-old's curiosity into our midst like a trump card in a hand of bridge.

In the same detached tone with which she might ask me to braid her hair, she now asked, "Grandma, are you going to die?"

I could see all the sets of grown-up eyes shooting shut-up-kid darts at her. Looking at my granddaughter, my instincts told me that this question had to be answered, and in a way that she could easily understand. I didn't hesitate. I had to pre-empt anyone who might want to deflect the issue. I replied, "I don't know if Grandma is going to die from this. But she's not going to die right away. That's for sure. Everybody dies sooner or later; you know that Amanda."

Heads now shifted in my direction, as if following the ball in a tennis match, and with the same collective trepidation. I continued speaking directly to Amanda.

"You like living next door to Grandma, don't you?" I asked.

"Yeah ..." she said, cautiously, wondering what this had to do with anything.

"It's kind of neat, isn't it? Now, if Grandma dies, she is going to heaven. And someone's got to get there first to make sure that when you guys arrive, we can all live on the same street again."

"Okay," Amanda said, shrugging her shoulders, satisfied. All present, except for one, exhaled in perfect unison. It was one of my sons-in-law who didn't allow himself this luxury, instead blurting out, "Could someone pass the butter, please?" Not a subtle stand-in for the real thing, which was, of course, "Whew. We got through this one."

Afterword

I should tell you that Dr. B. and I have remained on very good terms, and I always enjoy my office visits with his receptionists. Although he practices other forms of plastic surgery, his priority is breast reconstruction. He often asks me to counsel other women, to answer their questions and help them deal with their emotional issues. This is not much different from my work at Weight Watchers. I use my own experience to help others because I know what they are going through. And if anyone wants to see the evidence, I'm proud to bare my breasts. I've been doing show-and-tell for years, becoming Dr. B.'s one-woman hallelujah choir.

By the way, the office in the mall was temporary, while he waited for his permanent facility. He is in a new and modern medical building now. When you walk in, what you see is a reflection of his strength of character. It is not a Hollywood set; that's not his style. It's a place where good comes from bad and dreams turn into realities.

Before breast cancer, my life was a dream. And I intended to keep it that way. The moment I was diagnosed, I considered breast cancer an inconvenience, nothing more. And it was hard work getting my family to accept my point of view. They were often tempted to pamper me, to treat me like a china doll — the last thing I wanted. I had built up my resilience a long time ago, and felt comfortable with the person I had become. But I was afraid of hurting them. I didn't want my family to feel that I was rejecting their kindnesses. And, of course, there was a much more serious issue. Now that I, their mother, had breast cancer, my daughters were at higher risk of getting it themselves. So, even if occasionally I felt depressed, I couldn't afford to show it. I have always tried to be a good role model for my kids. Now this was more critical than ever. I had a responsibility to temper my daughters' fears for themselves.

Today, my weight remains a continuous struggle, and the more I get involved with breast cancer (I am also a Reach to Recovery volunteer), the more I realize doctors are unwilling to take that one step beyond "curing" you that would help women resume a normal life. Tamoxifen and chemotherapy have after-effects that no one wants to talk about. And I'm not only referring to weight gain. There is another, very delicate matter — a decrease in your sex drive. Does the medical community believe that we have no right to be concerned about the way we look, the way we feel, or about sex for that matter, just because we've had cancer? These inconveniences are not a "fair" trade-off, and I won't settle for just being happy that I'm alive. I want to be happily alive. And I will do whatever I can to help myself and others in my situation. My mission to save the world continues.

I thank the Lord that I have a husband who supports me in everything I do. We celebrated our thirty-sixth wedding anniversary last year. Quite an achievement, I think, for an old-fashioned sweater-girl who has lost both her breasts, and the man who married her.

Judy Reimer

Vancouver, B.C.
Date of Birth: September 18, 1957
Date of Diagnosis: January 8, 1990

When I see the last smile, hear my name for the last time, or feel the warm flow of life in a palm pressed gently into mine, when all this happens, I will quietly take my leave, content in my heart and soul that I have been blessed with beauty and goodness and love.

This is not to say that I've always had a privileged life, or even that I'm particularly grateful for the illness that has brought me all these things. I have also encountered indifference and lived through many painful disappointments. But tempted as I am to tell a tale of woe, I will try to make my story a celebration. To do so is more than a personal desire; it is, indeed, a mother's obligation. For when my children grow up, I want them to understand that good enhances life far more than malice could ever diminish it.

And so, my story begins.

***

The birth of my daughter, Louise, in September of 1988, was an immensely joyous occasion. With her arrival our family was complete, and, if only for a little while, I felt that the world held the promise of all my adolescent dreams. I was married to the man I had fallen in love with, had a career as a teacher in psychiatric nursing, a son, and now a daughter, a house in the suburbs, and a Siberian Husky named Leika. Everything was picture-perfect, if only for a little while.

After our arrival home from the hospital, I noticed that Brolin, my one-and-a-half-year-old, was not adapting well to our new family situation. Using his limited but unequivocal repertoire of tactics, he made it clear that he was not going to put up with this new little person in his life. Brolin was sure that we would change our minds and send Louise back to where she had come from. "Not such a bad idea," my husband joked one day, as he began to immerse himself in his job, working longer and longer hours, often way past midnight.

I, too, was committed to my work, and decided very early on that I would return to it just as soon as my maternity leave ended. Caught in the flow of the times, I readily opted to send the kids to daycare. Parents worked, children were cared for by others, and that was the eighties' way of life. It was convenient and quite reasonable to assume that everything would work out fine.

However, Brolin had problems from the very beginning. My niece had stayed home with him when he was born, and now he would have to accept two dramatic events in his short life — the loss of his home environment, and the loss of his status as an only child. At first I thought that his morning temper-tantrums were normal, that he only needed a period of adjustment. But the crying never stopped, and daycare turned into a horrible experience. Something had to change.

Eventually, after a lot of soul-searching, I decided to take an extended leave of absence from my job and become a stay-at-home mom. I had no concrete plans for the future. I just wanted my kids to be raised under the best circumstances I could give them.

I was very happy in the role of a housewife and never, for a moment, considered the job burdensome, but I longed for the company of adults. My sister and mother were living at the other end of the country, all of my friends were working, and increasingly my husband and I saw less and less of each other. As the months passed, and my ever-present feelings of isolation grew, I began to contemplate returning to work again. My work was not just a job; it was more like a mission, a life-long labour of love.

Growing up in a large family, I noticed, even as a youngster, that unresolved problems pain the soul, whereas meaningful communication nourishes it. So, once I decided to become a nurse, my path inevitably took me toward psychiatry. The mentally ill are our forgotten population, the underdogs of the patient community. And it was important for me to do a job that had consequence and merit, and gave something back to society. I never wanted to save the world, I just wanted to save people.

One quiet, rainy afternoon while the children were napping, I found myself lying on the sofa with my arms around Big Ted, my son's teddy bear, trying to empty my head of its messy bin of thoughts. But the moment I allowed my eyes to close, a distant memory claimed my concentration. I was standing in the lobby of the hospital, watching one of my long-term patients cautiously zig-zag through the crowd, seconds away from entering a strange, new world. We had just come down in the elevators together, and I had stayed behind to admire her. What a sight she was. Her shoulders were no longer hunched, her clothes were clean and neat, and she held her head high, perhaps deliberately so, because she sensed that I was still there. When the automatic doors opened in front of her, she stopped abruptly, and I held my breath. Then she turned around and began to wave, using the full length of her arms and both hands, like an exuberant child at the gates to Disneyland. I waved back and kept on waving as she passed through the doors and stepped onto the sidewalk, back into a normal life.

Suddenly, a frail voice rhythmically chanting "Mommy, Mommy, Mommy, Mommy," got me on my feet, and I hurried to check if my two precious babies were all right. With that, my daily routine should have picked up where it had left off. But I didn't bundle up the kids to take them for a walk. I made myself a cup of coffee instead, and sat at the kitchen table, evaluating babysitting options for Brolin and Louise. After the disastrous daycare experience, this was an issue I had avoided.

Over the next several weeks, searching for the ideal solution became a major preoccupation. Then, by a stroke of genius or maybe luck, everything fell into place. I found someone who shared my views on child-rearing — she had had a similar experience at the same daycare facility — and who also wanted to return to work, but only to a part-time job. I, on the other hand, mostly taught clinical nursing, which split my time between the Nursing College and the hospital. Twice a week I had rounds with my students in the hospital. On the remaining three days I did course-related work at the college, something I could accomplish equally well at home. And so the deal was struck. My friend, Louise, and I would alternate our days so that one of us could always go to work, while the other looked after the children.

I called my supervisor at the college and told her that I was ready to return. The first day of class for my new clinical course was set for Tuesday, January 9, 1990.

I rummaged through the drawers for a thick, red pen and circled January 9 on our kitchen calendar. Later that evening, after the kids were asleep, I felt a sudden surge of energy and began planning for the best Christmas of our lives. We'd have a real Christmas tree, full height, with some new decorations. I'd bake a gingerbread house and lots of gingerbread people. I'd dig out my grandmother's holiday recipes — my eggnog had never been as good as hers — and make the turkey stuffing from scratch. I'd place an order for a stack of firewood right away. On and on. The last item had a question mark beside it: will the children get a peek at Santa on Christmas Eve? To my relief, when I approached my husband about it, he actually agreed. Maybe things were going to start looking up on that front as well.

Days later, my sister called from Ottawa to tell me that the family were coming to spend the holidays with us, and I couldn't contain my joy.

Eileen is my only sister, and because we live so far apart I cherish the times I am able to spend with her. We fool around a lot and tease each other to tears. We gossip and reminisce, but mostly we just talk. Eileen's greatest talent is her discipline when it comes to listening to a voice other than her own. No doubt she says what she has to say, but I never feel as if she is formulating her next sentence while I'm talking, or that she is waiting for me to take a breath so that she can jump in and take over. Throughout the years, whether she was physically close or thousands of miles of telephone-wire away, I have always felt Eileen's genuine concern for me.

The incident that would permanently change my life happened a few days before Christmas. The women were all in the living room, a rather small place made cozy and comfortable by the presence of family, ever mindful of the little ones who were rushing about, each according to his or her own mobility. I was nursing Louise, Eileen was sitting cross-legged on the floor in front of me, humming along to Christmas carols on CBC-FM, and Eileen's mother-in-law was in the rocking chair by the window, assiduously knitting a miniature, pink sweater.

This idyllic hiatus from the continuous hustle and bustle of the house ended suddenly when Eileen jumped to her feet and began to chase after Brolin, who had eyed an open door to the basement and was deliriously running toward his tricycle at the bottom of the concrete stairs. From where I was sitting, I could see Eileen's outstretched arm reach the door ahead of Brolin's sprinting feet, and another vignette from toddler-life came to an end with the loud, powerful bang of a door and a forceful "Gotcha!" from a vigilant aunt. Two frustrated souls made their way back to the living room, Brolin using his body to show it, my sister making faithful promises to the Almighty that she'd catch the delinquent male who had left the basement door ajar. "This would *never* happen in my house," she roared. In the meantime, Louise had had enough and pushed herself away from me.

Using my best baby voice, I looked at Louise and said, "Do you want to go to auntie Eileen?"

"Give," my sister responded, arms bent at the elbows, her hands beckoning. I then proceeded to make myself presentable for mixed company again. I lifted my breast into my bra, and this was the instant I first felt the mass. I ran my fingertips over it, estimating the length to be about five centimetres.

My first reaction was that it was probably an inflamed milk duct. And as I continued to examine it, I noticed that the mass was quite mobile and didn't have any of the characteristics of a typical tumour. Besides, my breasts had always been full of lumps, so new ones never frightened me. They'd come and they'd go.

I assumed that Eileen had exactly the same breast condition, and I immediately thought of asking her to feel it. I wanted her to confirm that I was right, that it was just another non-threatening lump. As it turned out, Eileen did not have lumpy breasts, so she really didn't know very much about these things. Nonetheless, she was here with me now, not more than five feet away, and she was my sister. "Come and feel it, anyway," I said. Eileen, still cooing and grimacing at Louise, put the baby down and walked over to me.

First I heard a gasp, then something like "Oh my God," and my sister's sweet expression vanished. I was looking into wide-open eyes, intently focused on mine. Her tone was motherly and not unfamiliar. "Jude, I think you'd better have this looked at," she said. "Just to give you peace of mind. Or, let me put it this way. Just to give *me* peace of mind."

Later that day I phoned my doctor, and within five minutes I had both a date for a mammogram and an appointment with a surgeon. The mammogram was scheduled for two weeks hence, right after the holidays. I would see the surgeon four days later, on Monday, January 8, the day before I was to begin teaching a new set of students.

I marked the appointments on the calendar, thinking how quickly January was filling up: Thursday the 4th — go for the mammo; Monday, the 8th — see Dr. E.; Tuesday the 9th — first day of work!

Satisfied that I had the situation under control, I resumed my holiday responsibilities as if I didn't have a care in the world. My only concern was to guarantee a good time for everyone. There were ten of us in an eight hundred-square-foot house, and I was constantly on the go. I did, however, continue to monitor the status of the mass, always in the belief that my first impression would prove to be correct. Goodness knows, I had enough milk to feed an entire nursery during a full moon.

What a wonderful Christmas we had that year, abundant with memories of my own childhood holidays growing up on the Prairies. A modest house cramped with three generations of family, each involved in their unique preoccupations; plenty of food, drink and conversation; outdoor activities, making me ever so grateful that I lived in Vancouver, not in Swift Current, Saskatchewan; a warm fireplace; and presents galore. Through it all, our only disappointment was Santa's late arrival on Christmas Eve. One by one the children fell asleep, exhausted from the anticipation, eyes fixed on the front door. (That's where Santa will enter, I had told them, because the chimneys in Vancouver are too narrow for him.) In the early hours of Christmas morning, however, when the children saw Santa's presents lying in a pile under the tree, the night's anxious hours were forgotten.

Eventually, and to everyone's regret, real life snuck up on us again, and Eileen left with her family to go back to Ottawa. It was with a heavy heart and a brave front that I took them to the airport and watched them melt into the mass of humanity that was the holiday crowd, heading towards the security area and out of sight.

As soon as I got home, I decided to begin preparing for my return to work — there were only six days before my red-circle day — and, I suppose, this manufactured sense of urgency saved me from a dreadfully empty feeling. On Thursday, the fourth of January, the word "mammogram" was at the top of my list of things to do. Two weeks had passed since I first discovered the mass, and it had doubled in size to ten centimetres. I could barely feel where the mass ended and my breast tissue began. Still, I wasn't ready to theorize about a potentially serious health condition.

And the next day, Friday, I went into the hospital to get acquainted with my new environment. The hospital is a huge facility, and I had been assigned to a ward where I had never worked before. As I entered the building and stepped into the familiar lobby, I was filled with excitement, the type I used to feel on my first day of school after summer vacation. I stopped to look around, not for any particular purpose, but to indulge myself in the pleasure of knowing that I belonged there. Up on the ward, welcoming smiles greeted me. And, before I knew it, I was taking part in intelligent conversation again; I was being asked for my opinions; I became a member of a team dedicated to the same cause and speaking the same language. I left the hospital a richer person, valued and regarded as an equal adult. It had been a long time.

Then Monday came. "Judy, this is cancer," the surgeon said, "you'll need to have a mastectomy."

"Oh, dear," I replied, my thoughts turning instantaneously to my children.

"I'm afraid there's more," the surgeon said. "The tumour is too big for us to do anything." She stood up and reached for her coat. "As a matter of fact, you're going to follow me to the cancer clinic right now."

The next thing I remember was pulling my car in behind hers at the clinic's entrance where the oncologist was waiting for us. He hastily dispensed with the formalities, whereupon my surgeon left, saying, "You're in good hands, now."

The oncologist went to sit at his desk and began to shuffle some papers. "Beautiful weekend, wasn't it?" he said, without making eye contact. "Great skiing. Did you manage to catch the powder up on Blackcomb?"

What is he talking about, I wondered, as I watched him shuffle even more papers in my file. What on earth is he looking for? Surely he must know how anxious I am.

Finally, he began. "Now listen carefully, Mrs. ... Reimer. I don't want to scare you ..." He stopped abruptly and cleared his throat. "... but we have quite a situation on our hands." The oncologist went on to explain that because the tumour was already so large and growing rapidly, I would need immediate treatment to arrest its growth and — hopefully — shrink it down to almost nothing. I was facing three months of chemotherapy, followed by one month of radiation — to be administered twice daily — and another three months of chemotherapy after that. I wouldn't have surgery before August.

"When do I start the chemo?" I asked.

"Tomorrow afternoon."

"But I start work tomorrow," I replied.

"Well," he said, "I won't kid you. The treatments are not going to be easy, and you'll need to conserve your energy. I think you should give your work situation another thought."

Perhaps, in the back of my mind, I had prepared myself for a diagnosis of breast cancer all along. But his remark about work caught me completely off guard. I had been a driven person my whole life; duty resided in my very bones. Fulfilling a commitment, however large or small, was not a matter of choice. So, right then and there, I made up mind to finish what I had started. I wouldn't be the first woman to work while undergoing chemotherapy. Besides, it would be a nightmare for the college to find a replacement for me at this late stage. I couldn't let down all the people who were relying on me.

As for my dreams for self-fulfilment, for a personal renewal of sorts, I had traded those in long ago — if only one hour ago in terms of linear time — for nothing more ambitious than another chance at life.

"I take it you're married," the oncologist said.

"Yes," I replied. "As a matter of fact I called my husband from the surgeon's office, and he said that he would meet me here."

"Then I suggest we wait until he arrives," the oncologist said. "By the way, do you have any children?"

"Yes. A boy and a girl. Both under three."

"I see," he replied, stalling for time.

I felt very uncomfortable and didn't know what to do with the questions running through my mind. I didn't want to start off on the wrong foot. This man was holding my life in his hands. So I decided to join his verbal game of pitch-and-toss until my husband arrived. When he did, he headed straight toward the oncologist to shake his hand and immediately monopolized the discussion. How long would each session take, how frequently would I have to come for treatments, how long would it take for me to recover afterwards? Black and white issues, details, technical kinds of things which were not my priorities. Even today, after all that has happened, I acknowledge that these questions were valid from his point of view, but they were not *my* questions. I just sat there listening to the two of them talk as if I weren't even in the room.

The meeting ended when the oncologist left to see another patient. My husband drove back to the office, and I went home, calling Eileen the moment I stepped into the house.

She must have been anticipating something like this, because she didn't sound distraught, at least not as distraught as I had expected she would. We went over the same thing many times — that stroke, not cancer, was the killer disease in our family; that neither our mother nor any of her five sisters had ever been diagnosed with breast cancer. I was only thirty-two, I was strong and physically fit, the lump in my breast was new; therefore, in the end, everything would turn out all right. It was easy to be optimistic after a conversation with Eileen. She has a way of boosting, rather than confiscating, your energy.

I hung up the phone, ready to continue the rest of my day in a relatively normal fashion, which on Mondays included a trip to the library. I returned the books from the previous week and took out another half-dozen, all about animals. At home, the children sat cozily on either side of me, and we spent the afternoon roaming the animal kingdom — one of our favourite activities.

Time passed quickly, and before I knew it, the protracted dinner ritual was upon me. There was always a lot of cajoling to do. Brolin had developed a discriminating palate by then, and Louise was proving hard to wean. At least I didn't have to prepare anything elaborate for my husband and me. He usually ate out at night, taking a break from work, and I was satisfied sharing a modest meal with my son.

As bedtime approached, I did everything possible to prolong the activities with the children. Nonetheless, after the baths, Dr. Seuss, and a lot of hugs and kisses, the house became very still. I looked at my watch. It was only eight-thirty.

I had many good friends I could call upon in an hour of need, but Pam has always held a special place in my heart. Growing up together in Saskatchewan, we were inseparable. Judy and Pam, the Bobbsey Twins, sitting beside each other throughout high school, and later rooming together at nursing college. After my father died, when I was fifteen, Pam's family made a special effort to treat me as one of their own. I'll never forget a trip we took to the United States together. Twenty-five years ago going to the States was a very big deal, because Americans had so many things that we, Canadians, had never even heard of. In the annals of Judy's and Pam's private history, wiener-wraps took the glory on that particular trip. Of course wiener-wraps turned out to be nothing more than packaged frozen dough in which to wrap and bake wieners. But to two fifteen-year-old girls, the words on the box mesmerized us. We stood at the frozen-food section of the supermarket conjuring up all sorts of images — wieners, wraps, wieners wrapped and unwrapped — laughing uncontrollably, until I dare admit, we even wet our panties. When Pam's parents called for us to leave, we were frozen ourselves, each goading the other into uncrossing her legs and taking that first embarrassing step toward the exit.

On the phone that night, Pam cried with me, and the knowledge that someone else was sharing my pain made it much easier to bear. When she found her grounding — as she always does — she wisely directed the conversation toward pragmatic issues: what were the next steps in my treatment, how would all of this fit into my very busy life? She forced me to occupy my mind with tasks, which immediately succeeded in taming my more volatile emotions.

Indeed, starting that night, and for all the years that followed, idleness became my biggest fear. I knew that if I allowed myself just a crack of open space, my thoughts would rush in — the way Brolin had rushed towards that open basement door — and enter the part of my mind I was trying to place in quarantine.

9:15 p.m.: I was thinking that I had to look my best in order to make a good first impression the next day. I took a long shower, washed and blow-dried my hair, and went through my closet to choose the clothes I'd wear in the morning.

10:30 p.m.: I sat down at the dining-room table and began to review, for the third or fourth time, the notes I'd prepared for my first day of class. When I heard the front door open and saw my husband walk in, this time, I thought, maybe this one big time in my life, he won't let me down. And I immediately moved from the dining room to the sofa, expecting him to sit down beside me.

"I'm beat," my husband said, giving a quick glance in my direction. "I'm going to bed. And you should, too. It's past eleven. You have a big day tomorrow." He headed toward the bedroom. "Anyway, good-night," he said. Whether he didn't realize — or just didn't care — how much I needed him, I would only discover in the months to come.

The following morning I dropped the kids off at Louise's house and went into the hospital, according to schedule. I hadn't spent more than ninety minutes with my students when a colleague tracked me down on the ward, calling me away to an emergency. In acute-care psychiatry it could have been any one of a number of things. But when I arrived at the nurse's station, my oncologist was on the phone. He said that he had changed his mind, and rather than waiting until the afternoon, he wanted to start me on chemotherapy right away. "Please be here in an hour," he said.

For someone who believes that a dereliction of duty is a serious character flaw, it is hard to describe what this phone call did to me. However, I sensed that in the correct order of things, duty towards myself had to be at the very top.

I hurried back to the ward to tell my students that our session was over. "I'm really sorry about this," I began. "I can't tell you how badly I feel. Truly. I've never done anything like this before." But apologizing only made things worse, and it seemed that the more I apologized, the more reason I had for doing so. I should have made a clean getaway, rather than lingering and saying how sorry I was, taking upon myself the full burden of a wrongdoing that I had neither committed nor had control over. And I continued to apologize to everyone I saw on my way out.

***

There are two things I remember about my first chemotherapy session. One had to do with the reversal of roles I had to face. The other involved a box of chocolates.

"So this is how patients feel," I was thinking when I walked into the cancer clinic, now a patient myself. I had been a nurse for seven years, and the hospital had been my second home. But my experience didn't give me any type of advantage. In fact, I was very burdened. After having spoken with Pam the night before, and the medical staff that morning, I was aware of too many possibilities. What's more, my medical knowledge denied me access to a widely-acknowledged miracle healer called "hope." Hope and knowledge make incompatible bedfellows; one relies on belief, the other on science.

My second memory begins with the afternoon, after my chemotherapy treatment.

When the oncologist told me that the chemo had been moved up by four hours, I called my husband and asked him to meet me at the clinic. He did. And after it was over, he offered to drive me home. We were about to pass the fourth or fifth grocery store when I asked him to pull over. Chemotherapy plays tricks with your tastebuds, I knew that, but I didn't know why I had developed a sudden craving for chocolate. I stayed in the car while my husband went into the store, and within a few seconds I saw him come out with a small paper bag. I could taste the luxurious, velvety chocolate melting on my tongue. "Here you go," he said, passing me the bag. Inside was a roll of hard candy wrapped in cellophane. I hate hard candy. "This is much better for you than chocolate," he said.

Later in the evening, I was lying on the couch trying to recover from the events of the day, when the doorbell rang. It was my other dear friend, Carie, holding a two-pound box of Laura Secord chocolates. My eyes lit up.

"Hey, sweetie," I said to her. "What are you trying to do to me?"

"Well, it's like this," she said. "I've made some calculations. On this round of chemo, before your radiation starts, you'll have a session once every two weeks. That makes six sessions of chemo over three months. Right? So, it's easy. You'll have two pieces of chocolate after each session. And ... voilà! Two times six is twelve." She cut the ribbon, opened the box and ceremoniously displayed twelve individual pieces of chocolate.

"Yeah, sure, Carie," I replied. "That's only the top layer." I carefully lifted the cardboard in the middle of the box to reveal a second identical layer at the bottom. "So how do you explain *this?* Problems with your math?"

"Not at all," she said. "There are twelve chocolates for *you* and twelve chocolates for *me*. Oh, didn't I mention that I intend to be here after every one of your chemo sessions? You know. Just in case. If you need me, or something. So, Miss Perfection, has the mathematical mystery of a box of chocolates been solved to your satisfaction?"

We burst out laughing. Carie has one of those rippling laughs, short and quick, like a trumpet staccato that never stops.

We ate our two pieces of chocolate each, and as Carie closed the box, she showed me the top layer. "See. Only ten more to go!" she said.

If I measure time from the day that I was diagnosed, then I was born with a silver spoon in my mouth, my wealth defined by the generosity of those closest to me. I had always surrounded myself with friends, even before my illness, because my friendships were a matter of survival. I looked for, and was lucky enough to find in others, all the things I was missing in marriage. But in the years before breast cancer, my relationships had equal portions of give and take. After breast cancer, I could no longer give my share, and the less I was able to give the more I received. What can I call this if not true wealth? As for my two best friends, Pam and Carie, they were the twin diamonds in my crown of jewels.

Carie showed up one day with two twenty-four-roll packages of toilet paper, which, when placed one on top of the other, were almost as high as she was. "I noticed you were out," she said, "while in a compromised position." She'd appear at suppertime with a bag of groceries, feigning an English accent: "Dinner will be served at precisely six-thirty o'clock p.m. in the dining room." Then, back in normal English, she'd send me away when I tried to help. "Go lie down or something. Or go throw up. I don't care. As long as you get out of this kitchen."

An illness is messy. People cry. And Carie was always there, at the other end of the line, for an emergency or a laugh.

Pam lived in Regina, so she played a somewhat different role. She came to stay with me on two separate occasions, spending about ten days each time. The moment she'd walk through the door, she'd put herself in charge, taking on every conceivable task. She'd drive me to chemotherapy, read to the kids, make supper for everyone, clean the house, and pay the utility bills. On days when I felt like a human being, we spent many long hours over endless pots of tea, yapping until three or four in the morning, and even then not wanting to stop.

Saying thank you to soul-mates is effortless; give and take is a natural part the relationship. On the other hand, I had to learn to accept the generosity that so many others showed towards me during those first six months of 1990. My colleagues at the college put together a schedule to drive me to the clinic when I could no longer drive myself. They took up a collection to hire someone to clean my house. Sometimes friends would bring fully prepared meals so that I wouldn't have to cook. There was always a volunteer to take the children to the playground, or to babysit on the days that I couldn't get out of bed. I remember once, when I was overwhelmed with embarrassment, someone remarked that cancer is a community disease. It is the responsibility of friends and family to help, she said. *My* responsibility was to put effort and energy into getting well.

It would be dishonest of me not to admit that my personal nature was, perhaps, my own worst enemy. There is a Chinese proverb that says: "if you can't change your fate, change your attitude." But it is not a simple matter to rid oneself of life-long principles, and, cancer or no cancer, I had two kids in diapers to tend to (plus one on alternate days), a household to run, and an eight-week clinical course to finish. That I had underestimated what a horrendous load this would be became obvious only after my second treatment, when the drugs began to take a cumulative toll on my body.

Because I was dealing with grown-ups, the hospital was always manageable, regardless of my physical condition, and I could accommodate myself without compromising my students' training. We'd take unscheduled breaks and make up for them by adding extra time on at the end, or at the next session. If I couldn't last until the end of class, I would invite the students to call me at home, even on my days off. And, of course, everyone was nice and very understanding. Caring for three children in diapers, however, was a completely different story. Their energy levels and physical needs required more than my body's meagre reserves. By the end of the day, it felt as if I had no glycogen left in my body. I recently watched an Iron Man competition on television, and seeing participants crawl the last hundred yards on all fours brought back lucid memories of those gruelling babysitting days. Worse than any other thing, by far, was that horrible, suffocating smell. One bowel movement followed another, and another, and ultimately the day was an endless replay of the same scenario. I'd change a diaper and then run to throw up, twelve times a day.

The weeks and months passed, and the business of living became a day-to-day affair. Having fulfilled my obligation to finish my current teaching assignment, I wasn't so foolish as to take on another while still receiving chemo. At the same time, my friend, Louise, and I decided to end our babysitting arrangement. Life was about the now, and living took place in the moment. On my better days, when I should have just taken it easy, I forged ahead with my work, relentlessly preparing new courses and curriculums. I needed to keep busy and to feel indispensable.

Time and subsequent events, however, have given me another perspective on things. I now recognize that I was caught in a chemotherapy whirlwind at a time when my marriage was collapsing. Work grounded me; it was the only part of my life over which I had control. Buried somewhere in my subconscious, this may well have influenced my near-obsessive behaviour.

Whatever the case, the truth is that my good days made up for my bad ones — when my body was in so much pain that wearing eyeglasses hurt; when I felt the nausea launch an attack from my stomach, erupting at my throat like a volcano and sending me to the bathroom for the tenth time in three hours; when a chunk of hair the size of a grapefruit first stayed in my hand. Misery has strong powers of seduction. It tempts you to surrender to your better judgement and give up the fight. You hear a voice close to your ear saying, over and over, "it would be so much easier!" and you would sell your soul if you could, if only for an hour of respite from the wretchedness.

The positive attitude of the nursing staff helped me through my lowest points. I look at my charts today and know that there was very little doubt that the cancer hadn't spread. But their stance was that I was still curable, that it would be wonderful if they could hold me up as a person whose life they had saved.

With my chemotherapy behind me, I had the mastectomy in August of 1990, and two weeks later returned to teach in the classroom. I wanted to wait a few months before going back to the clinical work that I loved, until my immune system had recovered. But the course I taught during that winter would be my last.

***

Around the time that Louise was born, my husband and I had bought a piece of land in the Gulf Island chain, off the coast of British Columbia. Our property was located on an island called Galiano, midway between Vancouver and Victoria.

Galiano is only twenty miles long and seven miles wide, with no more than eight- hundred nature-loving residents. The rain forest and rugged terrain have remained mostly intact, and evidence of modern civilization is sparse. There are three small stores — with high prices — and five man-made parks. Our 5 1/2 acres of wooded land was situated at the top of a long, rocky road overlooking the valley.

Sometime in the spring of 1992, my husband and I began talking about building a prefabricated house and moving permanently to Galiano. How this idea really started is quite a muddle now. Maybe it was the counter-culture and easy-going lifestyle that attracted us, or perhaps some romantic notion associated with rustic living. Most likely, however, we saw Galiano as a last-ditch effort to make our marriage work, each of us believing — but never bringing out into the open — that a fundamental change in our lives would be the cure for all our ills. I didn't object to the idea.

Moreover, in the twenty months since my surgery, I had never fully regained my health and imagined that a pristine environment would breath new life into me. I battled the side-effects of tamoxifen, which were so severe that I stopped taking it. I developed lymph edema. The scarring from my mastectomy, combined with the heavy doses of radiation, limited the range of motion in my arm to about ten percent, requiring constant physiotherapy. And my immune system was still fragile. I hobbled from pneumonia to bronchitis to pneumonia.

Although I was working at the college, I had to keep away from the hospital because I was afraid of picking up other diseases. As for my husband, he was an electrician as well as an electrical engineer and believed, therefore, that he could establish a thriving business on the island. Certainly the demand for electricity was there. Galiano offered us a golden opportunity.

We sold our house, packed our belongings, and moved to Galiano in September of 1992. Our temporary home became an old, run-down, eight-foot trailer that previously had been the roof over our heads whenever we stayed on Galiano overnight.

At first I didn't mind living in the trailer at all. We fit right in with the old-time hippies who lived in buses and other makeshift residences. And it was a good reminder for me of how many things I'd had before that made my life easy — like indoor plumbing.

By December we were in possession of all the pieces required to assemble the house. We only needed to pour the foundation. Why my husband decided to build the garage first, instead of the house, I'll never know. But once the garage was up, we sold the trailer and moved in there, waiting for the rest of the house to be built.

The garage was a tiny place, and every square foot had to be used economically. The kitchen facilities included a small, two-burner stove, a half-sized refrigerator, a sink with four inches of counter-space on either side, and a small kitchen table. There was a bunk-bed and dresser for the kids, a two-door wardrobe for the grown-ups, and a desk for my husband. A plank on the wall, accessible by an eleven-foot ladder, served as our sleeping space. The outhouse consisted of nothing more than a hole in the ground surrounded by a wall of black plastic sheets, located at a distance of two city-blocks down the road. The shower was a garden hose nailed to the side of the garage.

My husband is a brilliant, charismatic man who knows electricity inside and out, but something about the way he conducted the business was not right, and we gradually found ourselves running out of money. By the time we moved into the garage, in December, the proceeds from the sale of our house were almost gone, and my only option was to get a job.

There was little available in terms of nursing on the island, so I accepted something in Vancouver, in a geriatric ward. It was casual work, meaning that I would go in only when called, but I took the highest-paying, twelve-hour night shift, commuting by ferry.

Galiano was still rather cold in March, and one afternoon, in my haste to run from the shower back into the garage, I tripped on a root and fell on my back. The pain was immediate and horrendous, forcing me to lie on the ground shivering, crying out for help.

I spent the rest of the day in relentless agony; there was no place comfortable enough for me to either sit or lie down. And as evening came, my heart began to pound, harder and faster, dreading what lay ahead. I had only one place to sleep and only one way to get there — by climbing up the ladder. Step by step, rung by rung, the muscle spasms burst like eleven separate gunshots in my back, until — one hour later — I reached the top and somehow managed to climb onto the four-foot-wide plank. That night I endured the worst pain of my life.

On the following day we called the local physician, who gave me some medication. I needed time and rest, he said. But the days passed and I had no relief. Early each morning, as I made my way slowly down the ladder, counting out loud the remaining steps to the floor, the pain was unleashed again. Then, by mid-morning, I would have to go to the bathroom, but I couldn't make it on my own. So I took a kitchen chair and leaned on its back all the way down the long, rocky road to the outhouse, stopping and starting, inch by inch, always in fear of losing my grip and falling. Then, back up again, at the same pace and with the same trepidation.

Three weeks after my fall, I was taken by boat ambulance to a hospital in Victoria, to try to have the pain stabilized.

Not maliciously, the oncologist said, "Go home and plant your garden, Judy. There is nothing we can do for you." The cancer had metastasized to my bones, and I had a tumour in my sacroiliac joint. The nerve compression and the interference around it were causing the pain.

I left the hospital two weeks later, in April of 1993, with a morphine prescription and a death sentence (one which I have appealed successfully during the past five years.)

This was when it became really hard to live. Although the pain was somewhat more manageable with the medication, all my basic life-sustaining activities were dependent on instruments of torture — the ladder, the plank, the outhouse, the shower. We had no money. The electrical business was at a standstill, and I had been obliged to quit my job in Vancouver. And, inexplicably, my terminal diagnosis brought out the worst in my husband's character.

Just before moving to Galiano, I had found out that not all of his late nights working had been spent in the office. Here, I didn't know what he was doing during the day. He wasn't getting contracts for his business, and he certainly wasn't building the house. The prefabricated pieces we had received four months earlier were lying untouched on our property. What grieves me the most, however, what still makes me cry, is remembering how often I told him, point-blank, that I needed his help. To pick up milk for the kids. To wash the dishes. To put a door on the outhouse. To secure the base of the shower — a three-foot-square pallet thrown down on a patch of bumpy earth — which terrified me each time I stood on it. When we actually had a conversation and I'd had a pain-free day, he would remark, "See, there's nothing wrong with you, Judy. What's all the fuss about?" Other times, when I urged him to use the proceeds of my life insurance to provide a decent house for the kids, he told me he'd rather spend the money on a sportscar. And twice his eerie nonchalance carried the words: "Why don't you just hurry up and die."

I used to believe that my husband wasn't really a malicious man, just a man in complete denial, someone unable to imagine what his future would be like and how he would manage with the children if I were gone. His denial was not tied to his love for me; I admitted that much to myself. It was tied to fear. Ultimately, however, my life with him had always been about the kids.

It was a time of deep despair. I rarely talk about this period of my life nowadays. I don't want to remember, and inevitably people find it hard to believe. Hindsight always puts a different perspective on things, whereas in the midst of a crisis we improvise, doing everything that we can to get through it. Sometimes we get lucky and our strength is bolstered by unexpected events.

Shortly after we moved into the garage, before my fall, I was woken up in the middle of the night. I know it wasn't a dream because I was sitting upright in my bed, my wits about me, looking at my actual surroundings. The incident lasted just a few seconds, as long as it took for me to hear, "You didn't die three years ago because you didn't *know* me." All of a sudden, I had a pervasive sense of being at one with the world, and from that night on I knew that my life and my little crumbs were part of a much bigger picture. This is what nourished my spirit on Galiano for the remainder of my stay. Lying in bed at night, when everything was very still, I could hear the wind coming through the treetops. First it was a faint, whistling sound, somewhere in the valley. Then it would gather momentum as it approached, louder and stronger, until I knew that the wild, roaring sound that surrounded me was my direct communication with a Supreme Being, whomever He may be, telling me that my trials and tribulations were not happening for nothing.

Nights, undisturbed by human voices, were always the best times for reflection, and one of my recurring contemplations was about the Holocaust. My dad had fought in World War II, and when I was growing up, the war had been a forbidden subject in our house. It stood in my mind as some awful, black, unknowable thing. Naturally, when I became an adult, I wanted to learn everything I could, and read voraciously about that terrible time. What fascinated me the most were the personal accounts of Holocaust survivors, people like Elie Wiesel and Viktor Frankl. I used to tell myself on Galiano that if other human beings had been able to survive unspeakable horrors, I could surely survive my marriage.

However, staying in the marriage made me, I am certain, the village idiot. Galiano is a small community, and everyone knows everyone else's business. They were well aware of the conditions under which I was living, and also knew about my diagnosis. I had joined a cancer support group as soon as I moved to the island.

Not unlike my previous experience, three years before, others seemed compelled to help me. And even if they were motivated by pity, they never made me feel it. They were honest, good people. At one of our regular meetings, in the summer of 1993, the group handed me a check for four thousand dollars, money they had contributed themselves as well as funds they had raised from the rest of the community — the church, the residents, the store owners — to send me to the Hoxsey Clinic in Mexico. It was clear that conventional medicine couldn't help me any more, so these wonderful people had made it possible for me to try this particular alternative treatment.

Then, one of my new-found friends decided that enough was enough, that it was time for me to move out of the garage. She scheduled a house-raising, organized down to the last detail, enlisting the help of more than a dozen kind-hearted residents. The house was assembled on a Saturday. One week later the roof was put up and at last I had a house.

I hadn't yet moved in when the island's minister paid me a visit. She came during the day, knowing that my husband would be out, and gently broached the subject of my marriage. I began to confide in her, although I continuously skirted the real issue. Finally, she stated exactly what was on her mind. "You know, Judy, everyone but you clearly sees what you need to do. Please think it over."

I told her that I *had* thought it over, that I had been thinking about nothing else, in fact. I would have left after returning from Mexico, had I not been worried about my kids. Working full-time was out of the question, so how would we live? How would I support my children? And what would happen to them if I were to die? By this point in our marriage, my husband provided virtually no support, financial or otherwise. What help would he offer once I were no longer his wife? Zippo. Nothing. This was my dilemma.

But by the time the rainy weather signalled the onset of winter in British Columbia, I knew I'd never make it through another month on the island with my husband.

My sister mailed us three plane tickets to Ottawa because I didn't have a penny in my wallet. And as the kids and I stood at the wharf, waiting for the ferry to take us to Vancouver, I saw an elderly acquaintance walking very purposefully toward me. We had befriended each other on the island, and I assumed she just wanted to say goodbye. But when she came up to me, she waited until the kids were out of earshot before pulling an envelope out of her purse. "Use this to buy winter clothes for all of you," she whispered. Inside was a money order for one thousand dollars.

Ten hours later, ensconced in the safety of my sister's house, I was both relieved and overwhelmed by the enormity of what I had done, and Eileen and I had a long, intimate conversation. It was the first time in my life that I revealed the whole truth to anyone. "There's one thing I really don't understand, " Eileen said. "You told me yourself, a month ago, that blood, sweat and tears went into raising that house on Galiano. Why on earth didn't you move in?"

Without even thinking, the answer popped into my head. "Because," I replied, "I knew that if I did, I'd never leave."

***

The children and I lived with my sister in Ottawa for eight months, which was a blessing, because my health had taken a turn for the worse. The doctors discovered tumours in my vertebrae, which were pressing against my spinal cord, and sometimes the pain was so intense that I simply wanted to die. Morphine wasn't effective enough, but a series of palliative radiation treatments turned out to be a tremendous relief.

When Eileen's husband was transferred to Kelowna in June of 1994, I decided to return to Vancouver. "Guess what, guys!" I said to the kids. "Mommy is feeling very well right now, so how would you like to take a long trip by car, a really long trip, all the way across the country?" I was so often ill, or bedridden, that I didn't want to squander any opportunity that would provide my children with good memories of their mother. They were old enough to remember this trip for the rest of their lives. Brolin had already turned seven and Louise was almost six.

They started jumping up and down, clapping their hands and yelling, "Yeah, yeah," their excitement swelling with every new item I added to the list of things to bring. But the real fun began with the purchase of a tent, three sleeping-bags, and other camping paraphernalia.

After seven days and nights of assorted adventures — including unexpected encounters with some of our story-book animals — we arrived in Vancouver, where we initially lived with my friend, Frances. About two months later we moved into a place of our own — the basement-suite of a house. I wasn't very happy being cooped up beneath the ground, but it was the only thing I could afford. Then the landlord decided to raise the rent, and I soon found myself studying the classifieds. Although there was a shortage of available housing in Vancouver, I got lucky and found a three-bedroom house within my means. Finally, after years of living like a gypsy, I would have a real home, and a good-sized front garden, too. Of course the house was also very important for the children — more for their psychological development than anything else. They needed their own space and privacy.

As soon as I signed the lease my friends convened a party, and over a long-weekend, we painted the entire house. (The colours were decided by committee, but the house was still beautiful. Clean and fresh and new.) And a few days later, everyone helped to move us in.

I had big plans for our first evening there. I wanted to make a fire, shut off all the lights, and pretend we were in the wilderness singing camp-songs and roasting marshmallows, the way we had on Galiano. Instead, I just lay in my bed, exhausted from the latest round of palliative radiation I had received, and the kids spent the night somewhere else.

One day, I saw a Sears truck pull up in front of the house. I went outside to tell the driver that he had the wrong address, but he checked his bill of lading, looked at the numbers above my front door, and told me there was no mistake. Five minutes later a twenty-four-cubic-foot freezer stood in my kitchen, paid for and sent by my former cancer support group on Galiano.

The quality of life with metastatic breast cancer is unpredictable. I could have a good day followed by a bad day, or I could have prolonged periods of feeling poorly or feeling well. Whenever the progress of the disease slowed down and I was able to manage the pain, I felt like a new person — almost like my old self — ready to become a useful member of society again. It was during one of these periods of wellness that I decided to see a career counsellor. I couldn't work in nursing any more, that was clear, but I was hoping she'd help me identify another field that might appeal to me. Something part-time, to supplement our cash flow. We certainly needed it.

Throughout my entire session with her, whatever area she'd explore with me, whatever exercise she'd ask me to do, I inevitably came back to one thing — that I loved fabric.

My mother is a talented, self-taught seamstress, and I used to spend a lot of time watching her sew. Of all the things she created with a needle and thread, quilts were my favourite. I was always the kid underneath who removed the stitch that got stuck.

I owned several books on quilting I had never read, and boxes full of material I had never touched. It was only when I became home-bound, after my fall, that I started to patch together my first quilt. I even took it with me to the hospital in Victoria, and thank heaven that I did. Quilting saved my sanity while I waited for that horrible other shoe to drop. In fact, when my doctors came to talk to me, I'd tell them to sit down and wait until I finished the part I was working on. This was my first step, I believe, in reclaiming who I was and, at the same time, securing the future role that quilting would play in my life.

I viewed quilting as a multidimensional metaphor for life, and once I was able to recognize the many parallels between my own life and the life of a quilt — from its inception to the very last stitch — the idea of somehow linking up the two began to formulate in my mind.

Foremost, I associated quilts with love — love for the person that a quilt is created for. For quilting requires more than artistic skill; it demands a very strong commitment, a tremendous sacrifice of time, and the desire to bring joy to another person's life. As a youngster, I watched my mother put her heart and soul into her quilts, over and over again, creating her unique folkloric pieces for every one of her children. Then, when I got ill, I realized that my life had really been a testimony to people giving a damn about me. And me giving a damn about them. A quilt seemed the perfect medium to symbolize that old-fashioned caring for one another that joins people together.

In the course of a "normal" life, lasting friendships and care among friends are all beautiful things; they enrich our lives. But in the context of crisis, these very same things take on more noble characteristics. I was virtually a single mother and had no family living close by. My friends made the meals, looked after the kids, and did all the driving. This type of practical support had made the difference throughout my illness, determining my quality of life. And now, I was thinking, if I cannot take this experience and somehow use it to help others in similar straits, I'm left with "good for Judy," and nothing beyond that. This was my epiphany of sorts, when the real focus of the quilt began to take shape: to develop a practical support network — of baby sitters, drivers, shoppers, house-cleaners and cooks — for women who do not have the friends I have been blessed with. The notion of "practical support" was not a sexy, newsworthy item, so I planned to use the quilt as the draw, raising money through individual and corporate donations. How, when, and where this would happen was buried in my mind, like a statue about to emerge from uncut marble.

I also had a very practical, financial concern. My vision — whatever shape it would take in the end — could not get off the ground without an initial investment on my part. And money was something I didn't have. In fact, I had never had a lot of money — perhaps the years preceding our move to Galiano were the best financially. But now I had no job, and making ends meet was worrisome. I was receiving government disability payments, and my husband, who was by then my "ex", paid intermittent child support — probably at the insistence of his new wife — but these amounts didn't even cover the basic necessities. One day a friend suggested I approach the insurance company that held my life insurance policy to try to get an advance payout of the proceeds. I knew that AIDS patients had seen some success in this area, but I had never thought it could apply to me. Well, it worked. They didn't offer me an overly generous amount, but with three combined sources of income, we had enough to live on. Not much remained for anything else, however.

Toward the end of my session with the career counsellor, she said, "Judy, I offer you my house and I want you to have a dream-night. We'll invite all your friends — and my friends, and their friends — and see if we can put all the pieces of your ambitious vision together. One person alone cannot make a dream come true."

Fifty people showed up for the dream-night and a pot-luck dinner. I began on a very personal note, telling everyone that I wanted to leave my earthly venue having created something of beauty, something that would endure beyond my illness. Then, not quite sure of the direction I was heading, I began to talk about my experience with this disease, and what friendships had meant to me, especially from the time I became ill. I explained how I envisaged the project connecting with that — how first and foremost, my objective was to provide women with practical day-to-day support. I also explained that I wanted to honour the many women who had died from this disease, and that I hoped to make this a grass-roots project, involving all types of communities. It was very important to me, from the beginning, that this not become politicized. There is too much energy wasted in the divisiveness of an "us" versus "them" attitude. People die from lots of different illnesses, and I didn't have any interest in putting breast cancer up against AIDS or any other disease. In my case it started in the breast; after that it's all the same thing. People are people, and pain is pain.

I bared my all, and revealed the intense urgency I felt to get this project underway, knowing that the remaining span of my life really was limited. I'd had all the palliative radiation to my hips that I could have, and my doctors were saying that if I got another six months of life, that would be great. Finally, I told them how the quilt actually looked in my mind — a scene from nature, with trees and wide open landscapes, and, above all, the wind. The wild and roaring wind that I had discovered on Galiano, carrying the voice of God.

The Life Quilt for Breast Cancer was born on that dream-night, on May 24, 1995.

It is actually a triptych, comprised of three separate quilts, or panels, each measuring 12 feet by 10 feet. The three centre pieces, depicting scenes from nature, were made by the B.C. artist, Gay Mitchell. They are 6 by 8 feet water paintings on cotton fabric, stitched to the batting and backing fabric with gold, silver, and bronze metallic thread. There are one hundred and thirty-six individual squares surrounding each centre piece, and every one of them reflects a personal story of love, loss, courage, or hope, honouring women's struggles with breast cancer.

More than fifteen thousand people, representing five generations — from an eighteen-month-old baby to a ninety-seven-year-old gentleman — have contributed to the stitching of the panels. The first two are finished and have been exhibited at over fifty libraries and galleries across Canada. The third is not yet complete.

Our initial support-oriented project will be the production of a handbook outlining strategies for newly diagnosed women on how to access existing resources. It will also contain practical suggestions for anyone who wants to help but doesn't know what to do.

Money hasn't poured in the way I had hoped. But now, with hundreds of people dedicated to this cause, I know that the actual network we envisaged on our dream-night will one day exist, whether I live to see it or not.

Afterword

At one time, long ago, I must have thought that I was a very powerful person. I was so driven that I took on many different roles and believed that the well-being and happiness of others depended on me. Ultimately, that type of thinking was pretty darn stupid, because it robbed me of the ability to discover for myself who I really was.

I'm quite different with my children than I ever would have been without this experience. I've learned that for them to have some disappointment, some pain, and some struggle in their lives isn't the worst that can happen. Today Brolin is eleven and Louise is nine, and when I look at them, knowing everything that they have gone through with me, I have no doubt that they can survive. They have had to move several times, and that hasn't killed them. They have had to do without. These kids are very good that way; they don't complain about it. In fact, it has probably made them much better people. I'm grateful for that. I'm grateful that the effect I have had on them will influence who they become as adults. I can talk about this now without crying, but I have to admit that I didn't get to this point without a lot of tears.

My hardest day was when I decided to buy them presents through to their twenty-first birthdays. I bought a variety of miniature crystal carvings, each of which has a special meaning. But, difficult as it was, it gave me a sense of release, because if something happens to me they will know that I was always thinking of them.

We don't become good sailors by sailing calm seas. I am a much more complete human being today than I was before my illness. And maybe I have finally grown up. I know now that life isn't about the glorious times — although those are wonderful perks. It is about being torn completely apart and, in the midst of it, having friends who support you in a way you could never have imagined. This is what fills a heart with gratitude.

If someone were to drop by at this very moment, I would invite her in for dinner. I feel terrific today, and I'm ready to cook up a storm. And if it were Carie at the door with my two-year-old godson, I would simply tell her, "Get out of my kitchen. Go throw up if you want. I don't care. Right now, it's my turn."

Also About Breast Cancer

Patient No More: The Politics of Breast Cancer
by Sharon Batt

"*Patient No More* is the best of both worlds. A moving account of one woman's immersion in the world of breast cancer as well as a carefully written critique of the breast cancer 'industry.' Batt exposes the intersecting interests of pharmaceutical companies, the class-bound world of fund raising and the research priorities that are funded ... It is impossible to read this engaged activist without a deepening understanding of the politics of women's health." — **Sandra Butler, Co-author of** *Cancer in Two Voices*

"A hard-hitting exposé ... *Patient No More* is one of the most comprehensive — and political — books ever written about breast cancer ... It concludes with the work [Batt] and others have done to unite women as a political force ... 'A new order is forming,' writes Batt, 'and activists are part of it.' For women with breast cancer, that vision of change may be the best hope."

— Maclean's Magazine

"Batt's book is the intelligent person's guide to this world of controversy and pain, an impressive and accessible example of investigative journalism at its best into a story that should remain in the headlines until breast cancer is routed." *— Ottawa Citizen*

432 pp   ISBN 0-921881-30-4   **$19.95/$16.95 U.S.**

gynergy books titles are available at quality bookstores across North America; ask for our titles at your local bookstores. Individual, prepaid orders may be sent to: **gynergy books**, P.O. Box 2023, Charlottetown, Prince Edward Island, Canada, C1A 7N7. Please add postage and handling ($3 for the first book and $1 for each additional book) to your order. Canadian residents add 7% GST to the total amount. GST registration number R104383120.